The Handmade Forgotten Herbal Apothecary

Over 250 Powerful Remedies at your fingertips

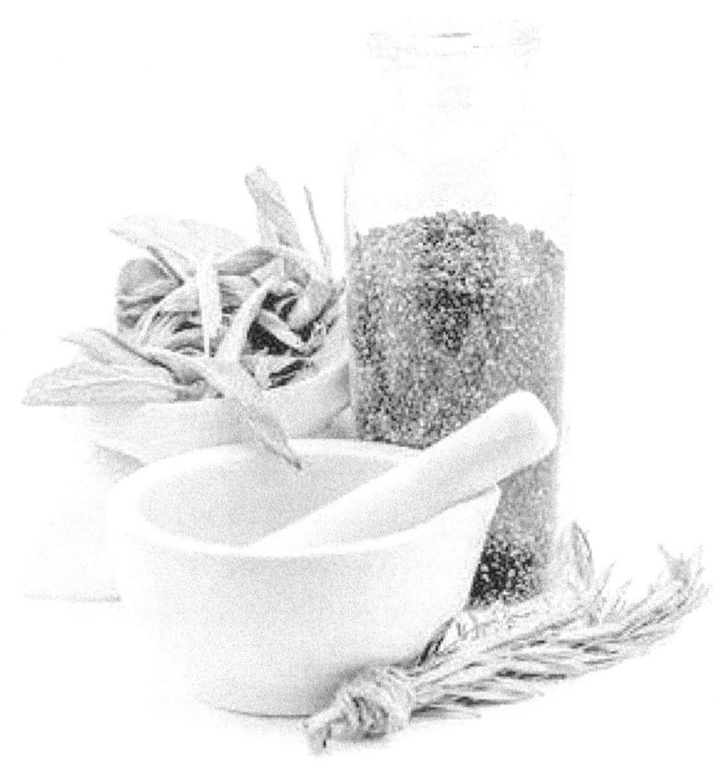

Dr. Martha Johnson
And
Prof. Asmyntha Gibs

TABLE OF CONTENTS:

Introduction:

A. Nature's Timeless Wisdom

Delve into the enduring tradition of drawing from botanicals and flora to foster gentle, comprehensive well-being that aligns body, mind, and spirit.

B. Cultivating Personal Empowerment

Gain the skills to craft your own botanical toolkit, tapping into the earth's bounty to maintain routine harmony and resilience.

C. Straightforward, Potent Preparations

Uncover over 200 user-friendly instructions for infusions, extracts, compresses, and ointments designed to enhance equilibrium and vitality.

D. Fostering Enduring Vitality

Adopt an eco-conscious way of living, minimize exposure to synthetics, and nurture ongoing wellness with plant-based supports.

Consider this volume your companion in embracing the earth's abundant treasures, delivering straightforward, reachable strategies for addressing common vitality challenges.

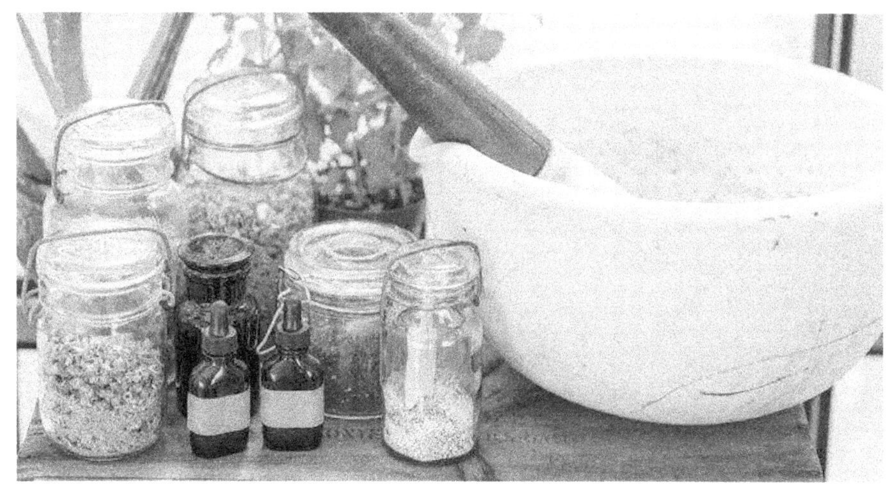

Categorization of Herbal Solutions

In this book, we've grouped the herbal preparations into specific themes centered around common wellness challenges. Every chapter aims to equip you with the knowledge to apply plant-based elements wisely and securely, fostering a deeper connection with your body's innate rhythms. Far from temporary bandaids, these approaches nurture sustained vitality, encouraging equilibrium, resilience, and intrinsic restoration. Dive into the details of each theme below.

1. Fortifying Immunity and Purification Building robust internal defenses is crucial for warding off everyday threats and maintaining vigor. Numerous botanicals harbor elements that enhance protective mechanisms while gently purging unwanted buildup, helping to avert routine ailments. Astragalus (Astragalus membranaceus): Valued for its adaptogenic qualities, this root helps fortify overall resistance and is frequently brewed into decoctions to support vitality during seasonal shifts. Garlic (Allium sativum): With its potent antimicrobial traits, garlic serves as a frontline aid against seasonal bugs, often incorporated into infusions or capsules to amplify cellular defenses and lessen symptom intensity. Burdock (Arctium lappa): This root excels in cleansing pathways, aiding liver function and fluid balance. Try it in a steeped beverage to flush out impurities, boosting energy and fortitude. Nettle (Urtica dioica): Nettle offers mineral-rich support for elimination processes, helping to clear pathways and reinforce barriers against invaders. Employing these plants for purification can assist in shedding lingering residues, heightening your natural safeguards and reducing vulnerability to disruptions.

2. Epidermal Vitality and Radiance Your outer layer often mirrors inner harmony, and various plants can calm irritations, temper swelling, and cultivate a vibrant, resilient appearance. Chamomile (Matricaria recutita): This gentle bloom eases sensitivities like rashes or dryness when blended into lotions or rinses, its mild aroma also aiding in unwinding for better glow. Tea Tree (Melaleuca alternifolia): Renowned for clarifying blemishes and balancing oils, tea tree extract is ideal in spot treatments to refine texture and ward off flare-ups. Comfrey (Symphytum officinale): Comfrey promotes tissue renewal for scrapes or rough patches,

commonly featured in balms to smooth and fortify barriers without residue. Evening Primrose (Oenothera biennis): Packed with essential fats, its oil enhances suppleness and diminishes fine marks, perfect for daily serums aiming at luminous, even tone. Weaving these into your regimen can elevate dermal resilience, accelerating recovery from surface woes and unveiling a more vibrant exterior.

3. Gastrointestinal Equilibrium Optimal nutrient processing underpins total harmony, with select plants capable of easing disruptions, nurturing beneficial microbes, and aiding the system's natural flow. Anise (Pimpinella anisum): Anise seeds help dispel discomforts like swelling or spasms, making a soothing brew ideal for settling after meals. Slippery Elm (Ulmus rubra): Known for coating linings to relieve irritations, slippery elm powder mixes well into porridges or drinks for sustained comfort. Licorice (Glycyrrhiza glabra): This root tempers inflammation and supports smooth transit, often used in chews or elixirs to harmonize absorption. Cardamom (Elettaria cardamomum): Cardamom pods stimulate flow and curb queasiness, a simple addition to warm liquids for enhanced breakdown and ease. These plant aids can realign digestive pathways, optimizing uptake and fostering a foundation for enduring internal peace.

4. Alleviating Aches and Fostering Tranquility Plant-derived options offer gentle respite from strains and worries, aiding in loosening knots and cultivating calm without synthetic interference. Arnica (Arnica montana): Prized for targeting bruises or overexertion, arnica gels or compresses help diminish swelling and hasten recovery. St. John's Wort (Hypericum perforatum): This herb eases nerve-related twinges and uplifts mood, suitable in topical applications or drops for holistic unwinding. Passionflower (Passiflora incarnata): Passionflower vines promote serenity amid tension, brewed into evening sips to dissolve worries and invite repose. Cayenne (Capsicum annuum): With warming effects, cayenne in liniments boosts flow to sore spots, providing targeted warmth for joint or muscular relief. Such botanicals deliver wholesome paths to temper discomforts, easing both corporeal and emotional burdens for a more centered existence.

5. Airway Clarity and Support Nurturing clear passages is vital for those navigating ongoing or periodic breathing hurdles, with certain plants excelling at opening channels, comforting tissues, and improving flow.

Peppermint (Mentha piperita): Its invigorating essence clears blockages, effective in vapors or rubs to refresh and expand airways. Osha (Ligusticum porteri): Osha root bolsters lung capacity against irritants, often in syrups to loosen buildup and soothe passages. Plantain (Plantago major): Plantain leaves aid in expelling excess, featured in steams or extracts to calm and protect respiratory linings. Elecampane (Inula helenium): This root encourages productive clearance for stubborn coughs, ideal in honey-based mixtures for deeper relief. These herbal supports bolster airway function, facilitating smoother exchanges and mitigating distress from environmental or internal factors.

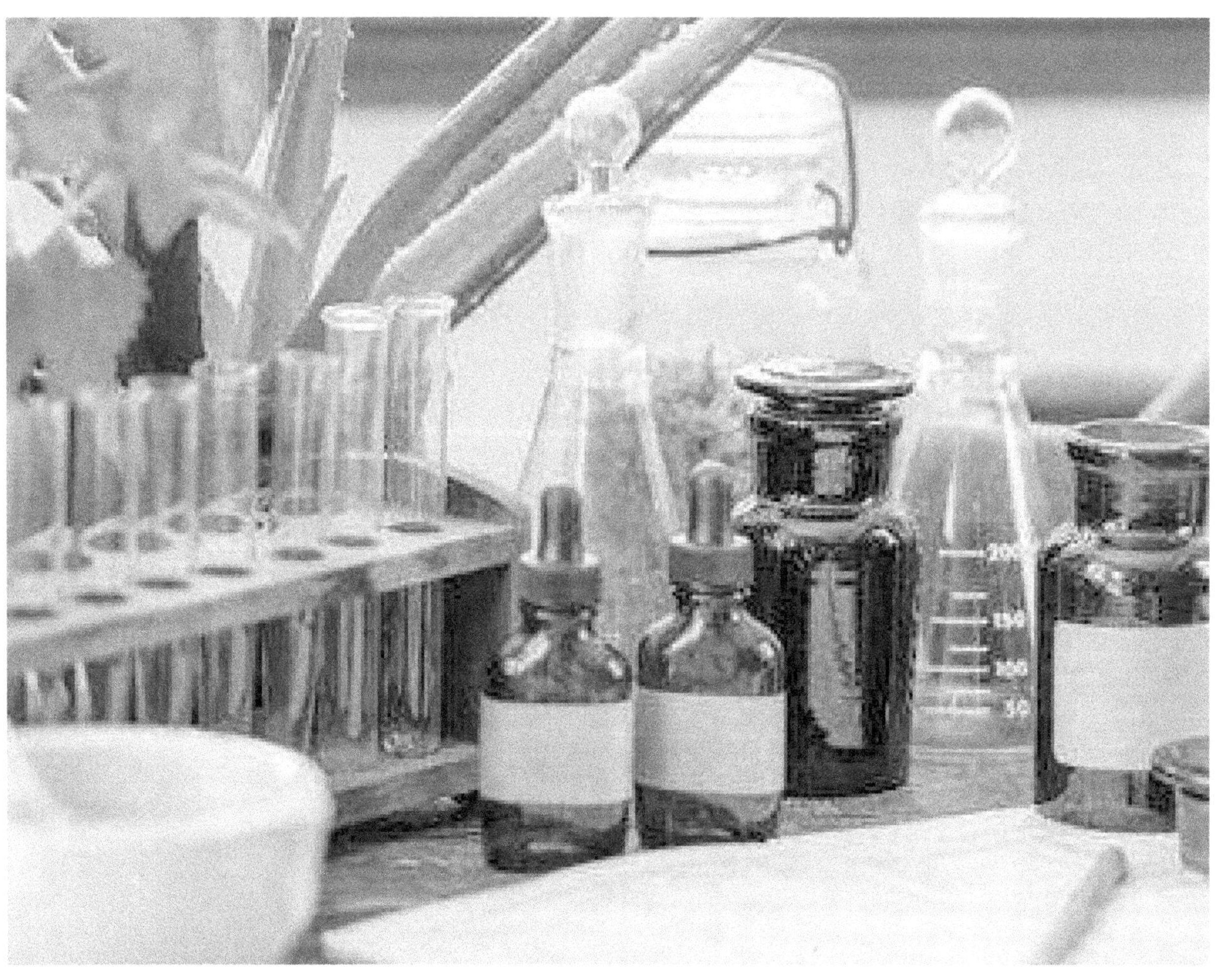

Building a Foundation: Investigating and Assembling Insights for Natural Wellness Formulas

Embarking on the journey of crafting or applying plant-based wellness aids demands a robust groundwork of inquiry. This exploration isn't merely about confirming benefits; it's the cornerstone for ensuring practices that are both reliable and beneficial. Thorough investigation underpins every formula, blending time-tested observations with contemporary understanding to foster confidence in their application.

Grasping the Value of Plant Potency

The essence of this pursuit lies in decoding how vegetation influences well-being. Vegetation harbors natural elements that interact with bodily systems, offering support for various functions. Delving into these elements reveals not only their potential but also the rationale behind their effects, allowing for formulas grounded in both heritage and empirical support.

Linking Past Uses with Current Insights: Numerous botanicals have been employed across eras in diverse societies. Examination helps connect these enduring applications to today's findings, verifying their ongoing utility while adapting them to modern contexts. This fusion strengthens the relevance of ancestral approaches in present-day self-care routines.

Key Resources for Exploration

The strength of your inquiries hinges on the materials consulted. Consider these core avenues for gathering dependable data:

Printed Resources and Scholarly Works
In-Depth Guides: Volumes dedicated to botanical profiles, such as those outlining cultivation, extraction, and application methods, provide foundational knowledge. They often include practical advice on proportions and forms, aiding in the creation of balanced mixtures.

Chemical Composition Overviews: Resources focusing on the natural substances within flora explain how these contribute to supportive effects. Understanding which parts of a plant drive specific outcomes informs thoughtful selection for various needs.

Specialized Publications and Empirical Reports
Scientific Periodicals: Outlets like those devoted to plant science and therapeutic applications publish analyses of botanical properties and tested outcomes. For instance, investigations into peppermint for digestive ease or echinacea for seasonal support appear here, offering structured evidence.

Practical Accounts: Examine documented experiences detailing how botanicals address real scenarios. These narratives provide actionable perspectives, illustrating applications in everyday situations.

Digital Repositories
Comprehensive Archives: Platforms aggregating reviewed studies, such as centralized medical databases, deliver detailed information on botanical reliability, interactions, and outcomes.

Academic Search Engines: Tools enabling access to scholarly articles facilitate discovery of recent explorations into plant elements and their uses, often with open resources for deeper dives.

Assessing Reliability in Materials

The trustworthiness of gathered information stems from source integrity. Distinguishing between personal stories and verified data is key to sound conclusions.

Author Expertise: Investigate the background of contributors. Do they hold recognized knowledge in fields like botany or wellness? Materials from established specialists lend weight.
Reviewed Content: Favor pieces vetted by field experts, as this process ensures precision. Avoid unverified online entries or informal accounts that lack scrutiny.

Verification Across Origins: Compare details from multiple trusted outlets. Consensus among them bolsters confidence, whereas isolated claims warrant skepticism.

Prioritizing Wellness and Risk Awareness

Caution remains paramount in botanical applications. Probing potential hazards and side effects is vital for developing secure options.

Risk Profiles: Determine if a plant poses any known concerns. For example, certain roots might affect organ function with prolonged internal use, while others could influence vitality levels. Associations or dedicated texts on plant safety offer extensive details.
Compatibility with Other Substances: Botanicals may alter the impact of common aids. Peppermint, for instance, might interact with certain digestive supports, and adaptogens could influence energy regulators. Studies in reliable journals highlight these dynamics.

Appropriate Application: Explore optimal preparation and intake methods. Variations in form—infusions, encapsulations, or external applications—affect strength and suitability. Establishing suitable amounts prevents overexposure.

Decoding Core Elements and Their Impacts

Central to inquiry is pinpointing the vital components in flora, which dictate their supportive roles.

Natural Substances: Key groups like antioxidants, volatiles, and stabilizers underpin effects. Antioxidants in berries, for example, combat stress, while calming agents in flowers promote relaxation.
How They Function: Investigate bodily interactions. A compound in roots might soothe tension by modulating response pathways.

Combined Effects: Certain pairings amplify benefits. Combining a spice with an enhancer, for instance, can improve absorption. Studying these interactions leads to more potent blends.

Real-World Applications and Structured Tests

Documented experiences and rigorous evaluations confirm practical value.

Individual Narratives: Review accounts of botanical use in specific contexts, revealing everyday effectiveness.

Controlled Evaluations: High-quality assessments, particularly those with balanced groups, provide strong backing. Tests on adaptogens for vitality, for example, demonstrate measurable improvements.

Cultural Botanical Insights

Exploring how communities have utilized flora uncovers lesser-known approaches, enriching modern practices.

Societal Traditions: Discover regional methods for addressing common concerns. For instance, berries have long supported respiratory health in some groups, now examined for broader relevance.

Generational Wisdom: Collect insights from enduring practices, detailing preparation and roles in well-being.

Ensuring Quality in Botanical Materials

Authenticity directly affects outcomes. Verifying sources guarantees purity.

Procurement Practices: Seek botanicals from ethical growers, favoring those without additives and harvested responsibly. Providers should detail origins.

Recognition Skills: Master identification to avoid confusion with similar varieties. Guides and educational programs enhance accuracy.

Crafting Balanced Mixtures

Using insights to design accessible preparations, such as liquids, topicals, or blends.

Liquid Extracts: Examine solvent-based techniques and ratios to optimize extraction, ensuring retention of beneficial traits.

External Preparations: Infuse elements into bases like nut oils to create soothing applications. Understanding absorption aids in effective design.

Recording and Structuring Discoveries

Maintain detailed notes throughout to streamline organization.

Personal Logs: Track findings, including observations and ideas, in accessible formats.

Management Systems: Employ tools to catalog references, facilitating easy retrieval.

Integrating Heritage in Contemporary Practices

Enduring insights from various societies validate many botanicals, tested through observation. These offer a lens for adapting historical methods to current needs, like using calming flora for modern stress relief.

Teamwork Across Disciplines

Collaboration between areas like plant science, chemistry, and health enhances understanding. This approach balances heritage with analysis, ensuring comprehensive formulas. Working with practitioners refines applications, considering interactions and forms.

Pathways to Empirical Confirmation

Structured tests bridge tradition and evidence. Well-designed evaluations clarify benefits and limits, with protocols ensuring repeatability. For example, berry assessments show support for seasonal challenges.

Risk Management in Plant Use

Balancing potency with caution involves studying both advantages and drawbacks. Some flora may cause unrest or pressure changes with excess. Beginning modestly allows monitoring responses.

Worldwide Shifts Toward Natural Approaches

Interest in plant-based options grows as individuals seek holistic paths. This trend expands inquiry, meeting needs for backed alternatives. Integrating with standard care enhances outcomes for ongoing concerns.

Eco-Conscious Practices

Responsible use preserves resources. Favor mindful collection to protect diversity, opting for home-grown or nearby options to minimize impact.

Connecting Heritage and Analysis

Studying communal plant uses reveals valuable methods, merging observation with study. This uncovers potential for diverse needs, expanding the scope of supportive options.

Archiving and Disseminating Insights

Detailed records build a shared foundation. Curating data on uses and profiles fosters collaboration. Contributing through various channels advances collective understanding.

To solidify the reliability of featured options, draw on strong backing from trusted avenues. This encompasses:

1. Structured Evaluations: Reference balanced tests demonstrating outcomes. Berry studies, for instance, confirm aid in shortening discomfort periods, while root inquiries support vitality.
2. Specialist Perspectives: Incorporate views from field leaders to build trust, emphasizing ethical and informed approaches.
3. Usage and Caution Details: Outline amounts, possible reactions, and incompatibilities. A root for calm might induce sleepiness, requiring care with similar aids.
4. Blending Legacy and Evidence: Connect historical roles with current validations, like floral uses for ease in various forms.
5. Ongoing Assessments: Include extended observations to affirm sustained benefits, supporting choices for lasting concerns.

This integration creates a balanced resource, aligning enduring options with verified insights for assured, practical use.

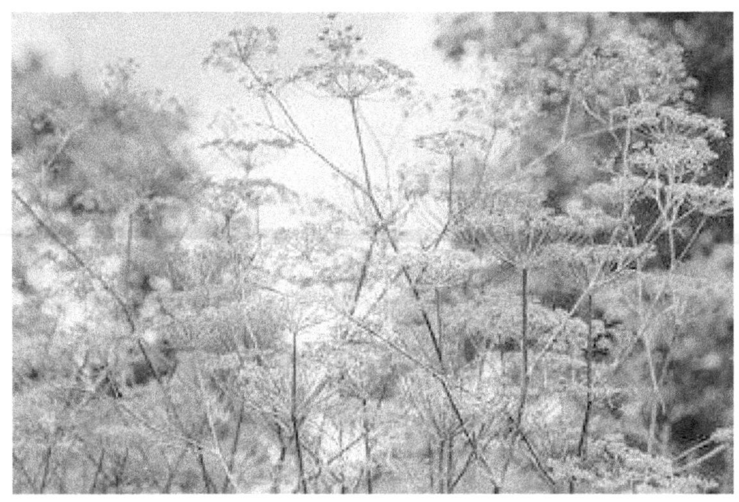

Harmony Herbal Infusion for Steady Hormones

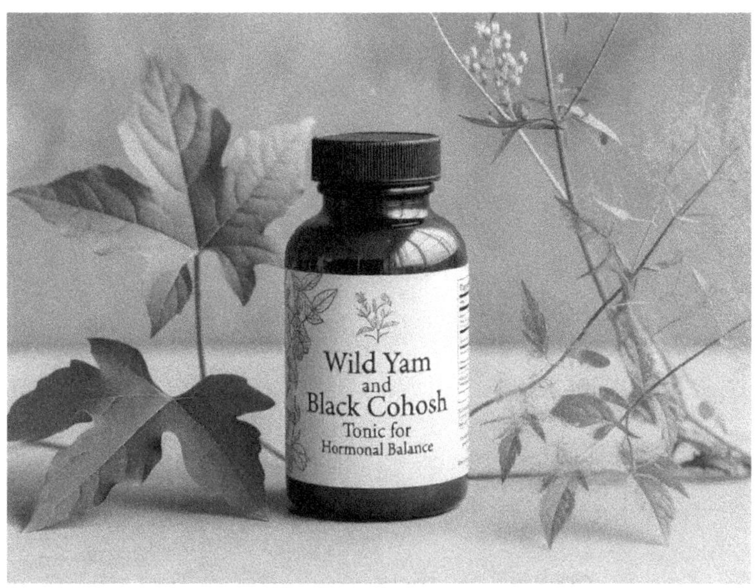

What You'll Need:

- 2 teaspoons of dried yam tuber
- 2 teaspoons of dried cohosh rhizome
- 4 cups of fresh water
- A dash of natural sweetener like maple syrup, if you prefer a milder taste

Steps to Prepare:

1. Place the yam tuber and cohosh rhizome into a saucepan and pour in the water.
2. Heat the mixture until it starts bubbling vigorously, then lower the flame to keep it gently cooking for about 15 minutes.
3. Pour the brew through a fine mesh to separate out the plant parts.
4. Mix in your chosen sweetener while it's still warm, if using.

Suggested Usage:

Take a small glassful each morning, especially helpful when dealing with changes like midlife shifts or monthly ups and downs.

Important Cautions:

Avoid this if you're expecting a baby or nursing. It could affect treatments for hormones or family planning pills, so check with a health expert first.

Calming Respiratory Blend Syrup

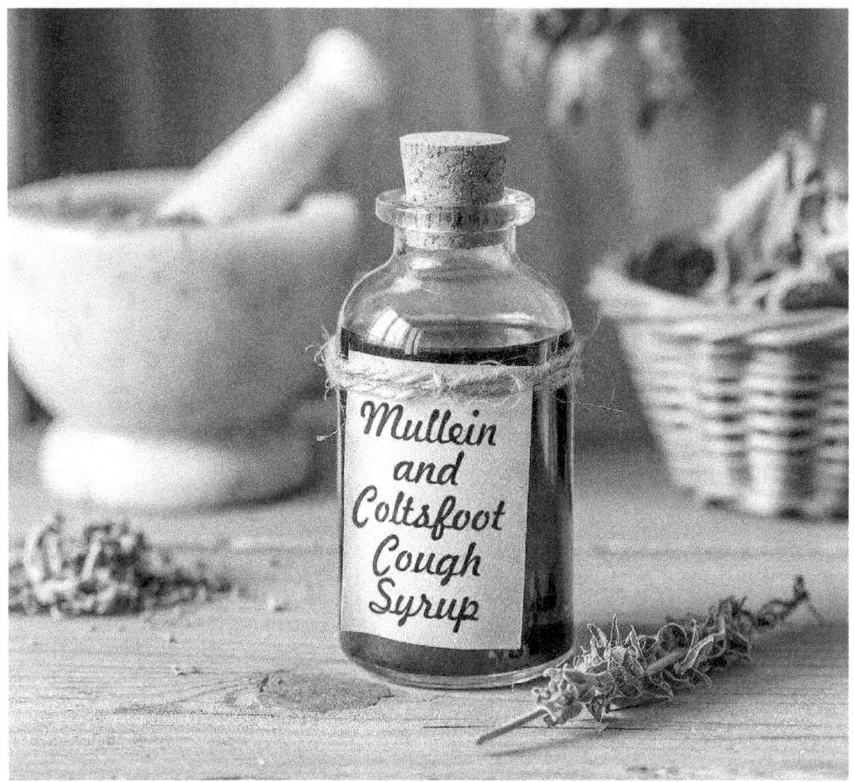

What You'll Need:
- 2 teaspoons of dried mullein leaves
- 2 teaspoons of dried thyme leaves
- 1.5 cups of fresh water
- 1/3 cup of raw honey
- 2 teaspoons of fresh lemon juice

Steps to Prepare:
1. Pour the water into a small pot and heat it until it just starts to bubble.
2. Toss in the mullein and thyme, then turn off the heat right away.
3. Cover the pot and allow the herbs to soak quietly for about 25 minutes to draw out their goodness.
4. Pour the liquid through a fine mesh strainer into a clean bowl, pressing lightly on the herbs to release extra flavor, and set it aside to reach room temperature.
5. Gently mix in the honey and lemon juice until everything blends smoothly.
6. Transfer to a clean glass container with a tight lid and keep it chilled.

Suggested Usage:

Spoon out 1 teaspoon whenever needed for throat comfort, up to four times throughout the day. It's best enjoyed at room temperature or slightly warmed for a soothing effect.

Helpful Precautions:

Always check with a healthcare provider before trying new herbal blends, especially if you have ongoing health conditions or are expecting. Skip this for little ones under 1 year old because of the honey. If you notice any unusual reactions, stop using it and seek advice.

Herbal Defense Brew with Coneflower and Flowering Herb

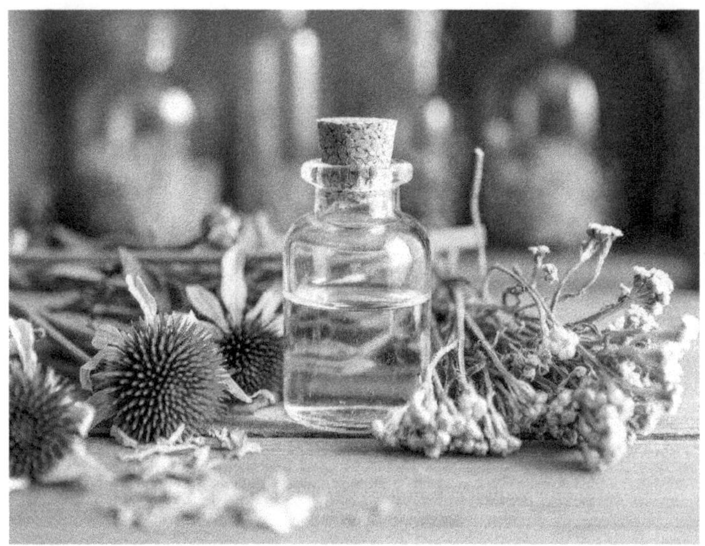

What You'll Need:

- 2 teaspoons of dried coneflower roots (also known as echinacea)
- 1 teaspoon of dried flowering tops from the achillea plant (commonly called yarrow)
- 1 small piece of fresh ginger, about the size of your thumb, sliced thin
- 2 cups of hot water, just off the boil
- A squeeze of fresh lemon juice (from half a lemon)

Steps to Prepare:

1. Add the coneflower roots, achillea tops, and ginger slices to a heat-safe mug or small pot.
2. Gently pour the hot water over everything and place a lid or plate on top to keep the warmth in.
3. Allow it to sit and infuse for about 15 minutes to draw out the natural benefits.
4. Pour through a fine mesh strainer into your cup, then mix in the lemon juice for a bright flavor.

Suggested Usage:

Sip on one mug each day to help strengthen your body's natural defenses, particularly when sniffles or seasonal bugs are going around. This warm drink can be a comforting routine to keep you feeling resilient.

Important Cautions:

Some people with allergies to plants like asters or chrysanthemums might experience skin irritation or other reactions. Avoid this if you have conditions where your immune system attacks itself, and always check with a doctor first if you're unsure.

Comforting Herb Infusion for Joint Ease

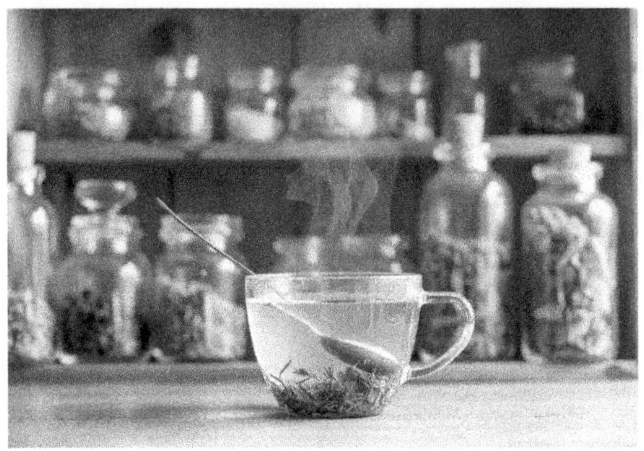

What You'll Need:

- 2 teaspoons of dried horsetail stems
- 2 teaspoons of dried nettle foliage
- 16 ounces of fresh water
- A dash of citrus extract, like from a fresh lemon, to brighten the taste

Steps to Prepare:

1. Mix the horsetail stems and nettle foliage together in a heat-safe container or mug with a strainer.
2. Heat the water until it's steaming hot, then pour it over the plant mix.
3. Cover and allow the blend to infuse quietly for about 12 minutes to draw out the helpful elements.
4. Pour through a fine mesh to remove the solids, then stir in the citrus if you like a tangy note.

Suggested Routine:

Enjoy a warm cup once or twice daily as part of your wellness habits to encourage joint comfort and soothe minor puffiness.

Important Cautions:

Skip this if you deal with any kidney concerns, since horsetail might strain those organs when taken in excess. It's best avoided by those who are expecting a baby or nursing. Always check with a health expert if you're unsure about trying new plant-based options.

Stress-Busting Herbal Infusion

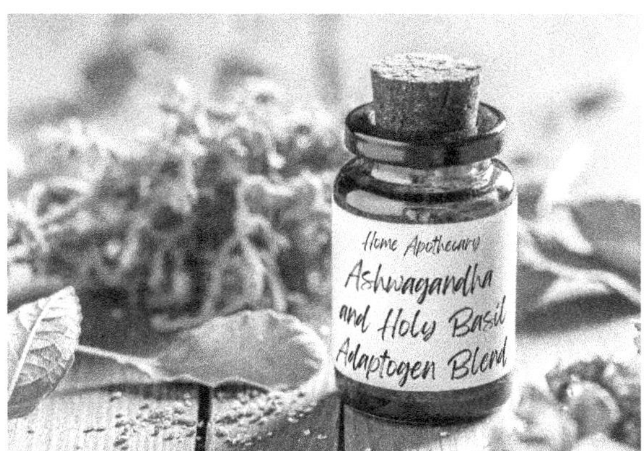

What You'll Need:

- 1 small spoonful of ground ashwagandha root
- 1 small spoonful of dried tulsi leaves (also called holy basil)
- 8 ounces of boiling water
- A dash of natural sweetener like maple syrup, if you want (optional)

Steps to Prepare:

1. Place the ground root and leaves into a heat-safe cup or teapot.
2. Pour the boiling water over the mixture and give it a gentle stir.
3. Cover and allow it to sit for 6 to 8 minutes to draw out the flavors.
4. Pour through a fine mesh strainer into your drinking mug, then mix in the sweetener if using.

Suggested Usage:

Sip on one serving first thing after waking up to help ease tension and lift your daily vitality.

Important Cautions:

Steer clear during pregnancy, since ashwagandha could potentially affect the muscles in the uterus.

It's best avoided by those with conditions where the body's defense system turns against itself.

Calming Herbal Infusion with Licorice and Marshmallow

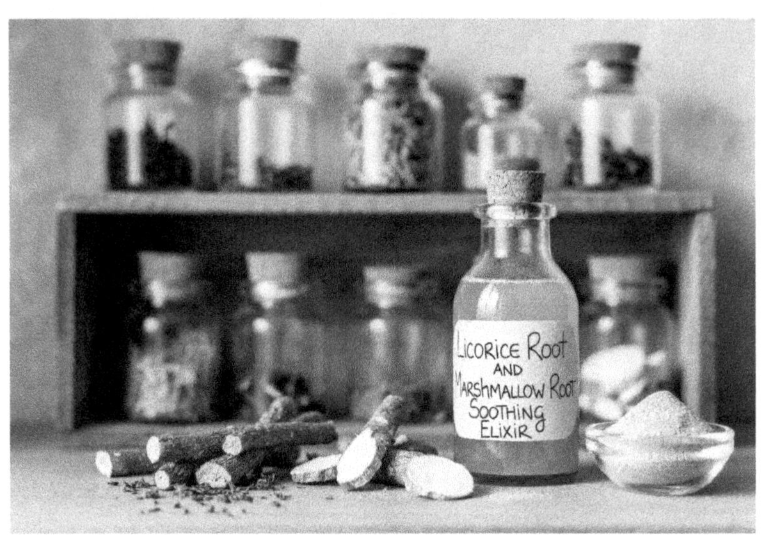

What You'll Need:

2 teaspoons chopped dried licorice root

2 teaspoons shredded dried marshmallow root

16 ounces clean water

A spoonful of natural sweetener, such as agave nectar or raw honey

Steps to Prepare:

1. Put the licorice and marshmallow pieces into a small cooking pot.
2. Cover them with the water and warm it up until small bubbles form around the edges.
3. Turn down the flame to keep it at a gentle bubble for around 15 to 25 minutes.
4. Take it off the stove, pour through a fine mesh to remove the bits, and stir in the sweetener while it's still warm.

Suggested Usage:

Take about half a cup, two or three times throughout the day, to help calm an irritated throat and promote easy digestion.

Important Cautions:

Skip licorice if you deal with high blood pressure, since overdoing it might push your levels up.

Marshmallow is generally fine in small amounts, but it could slow how your body absorbs pills, so wait at least an hour after taking any meds.

Calming Roll-On Blend for Nervous Tension

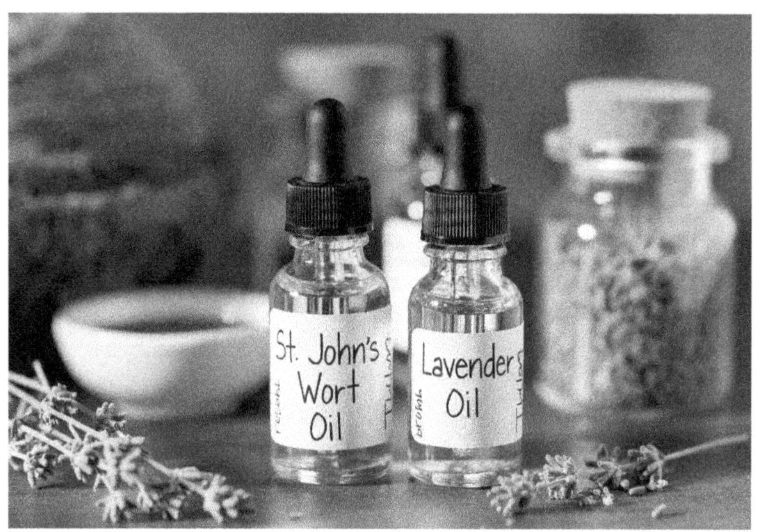

What You'll Need:

8 drops lavender essential oil

12 drops St. John's Wort essential oil

1 tablespoon base oil (like sweet almond or grapeseed oil)

A small roller bottle

Steps to Prepare:

1. Start by adding the base oil to the roller bottle.
2. Carefully drop in the lavender and St. John's Wort oils.
3. Snap on the roller top and lid securely.
4. Give it a good roll between your hands to blend everything together.

Suggested Usage:

Apply by rolling a light layer onto pulse points such as the inner forearms, sides of the forehead, or base of the skull during moments of unease or worry.

Important Cautions:

This mix could affect how some prescriptions work, particularly those for mood support or that impact brain chemicals like serotonin—talk to a doctor before trying it.

Limit time in the sun or under bright lights right after applying, since St. John's Wort might make your skin react more easily to rays.

Soothing Herbal Tea Blend for Tummy Comfort

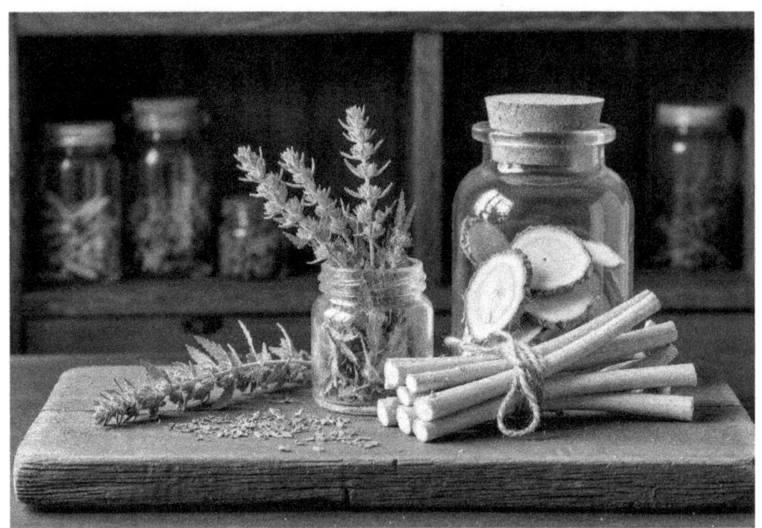

What You'll Need:

- 1 spoonful of dried mugwort leaves
- 1 spoonful of dried angelica root pieces
- 2 cups of fresh water
- A dash of natural sweetener like maple syrup (if you want it milder)

Steps to Prepare:

1. Add the mugwort leaves and angelica root pieces to a small pot.
2. Pour in the water and heat it gently until it starts to bubble lightly.
3. Let it sit on low heat for about 10-15 minutes to draw out the goodness.
4. Pour through a fine mesh to remove the bits, and stir in sweetener if using.

Suggested Usage:

Sip on half a cup about 20 minutes prior to eating to help ease stomach upset and reduce that full, gassy feeling.

Important Cautions:

Skip this if you're expecting a baby or nursing. Stay away if you've had issues with your reproductive system in the past. Always chat with a doctor before trying new herbs, especially if you take medications.

Tulsi and Lemon Balm Defense Boost Infusion

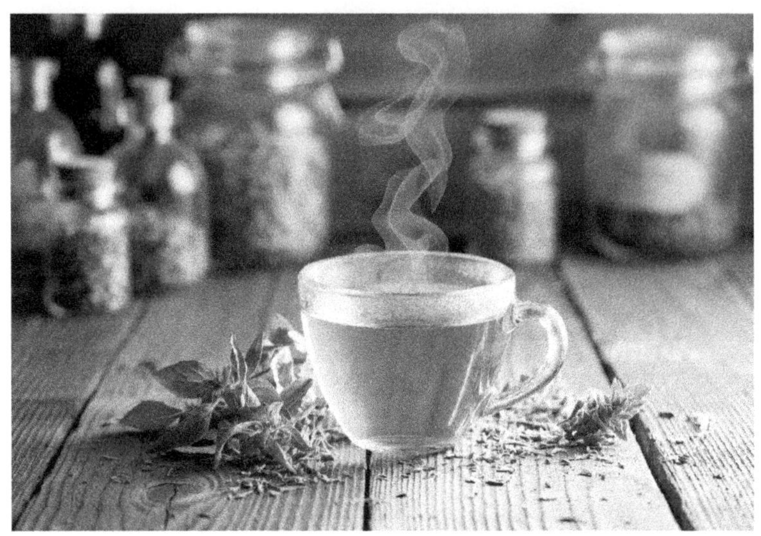

What You'll Need:

1 tablespoon dried tulsi leaves

1 tablespoon dried lemon balm leaves

2 cups fresh water

1 teaspoon raw honey (optional)

Steps to Prepare:

1. Heat the water until it reaches a full boil in a small saucepan.
2. Stir in the tulsi and lemon balm leaves.
3. Take the pan off the heat, cover it, and allow the mixture to sit for about 10 to 12 minutes to draw out the flavors.
4. Pour through a fine mesh strainer into your favorite mug, and mix in honey for a touch of natural sweetness if you prefer.

Suggested Usage:

Sip on one or two cups each day to help bolster your body's natural resistance and promote a sense of calm during busy times.

Important Cautions:

Steer clear if you're sensitive to plants from the mint group or have had thyroid concerns in the past.

Chaga and Reishi Mushroom Stress-Balancing Brew

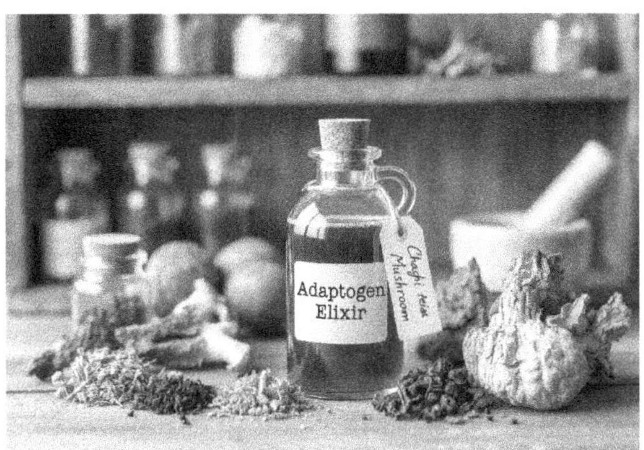

What You'll Need:

- 1 tablespoon of ground chaga mushroom
- 1 tablespoon of ground reishi mushroom
- 2 cups of boiling water
- 1 teaspoon of natural sweetener like honey or agave nectar

Steps to Prepare:

1. Mix the ground mushrooms into the boiling water.
2. Give it a good mix and allow it to sit for about 10 minutes to draw out the flavors.
3. Pour through a fine mesh to remove any bits, then add your chosen sweetener to taste.

Suggested Usage:

Sip on one cup daily to help support your body's natural defenses and promote a sense of calm and vitality.

Important Cautions:

People with weakened immune systems should skip this, as these mushrooms may ramp up immune activity in ways that aren't suitable.

Calming Kava and Mint Infusion

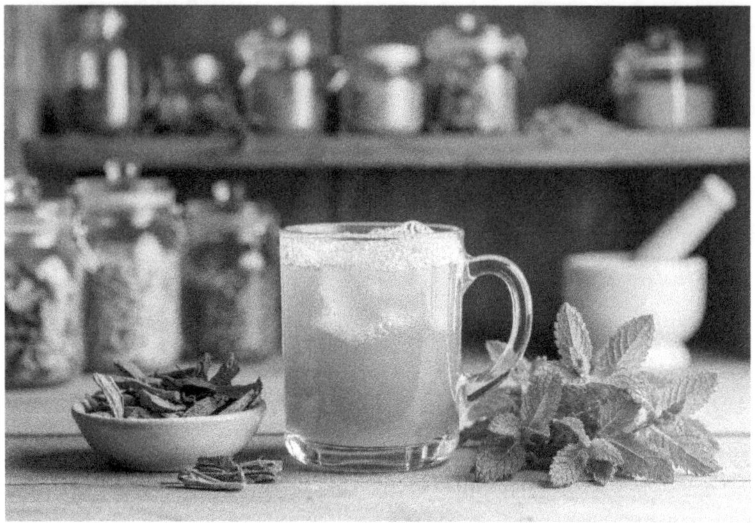

What You'll Need:

- 2 teaspoons of ground kava root (dried)
- ½ teaspoon of mint leaves (dried)
- 2 cups of boiling water
- A dash of natural sweetener like honey (about ½ teaspoon)

Steps to Prepare:

1. Place the kava root and mint leaves into a heat-safe container or mug.
2. Pour the boiling water over the herbs and let them soak for 8-12 minutes to draw out their soothing qualities.
3. Filter out the plant bits using a fine mesh or cloth, then stir in the sweetener if you like a touch of sweetness.

Suggested Usage:

Sip on one mug each day to help ease feelings of worry or tension.

Important Cautions:

Stay away from this if you've had issues with your liver in the past. It's best not to mix it with drinks containing alcohol.

Brain-Sharpening Herbal Blend

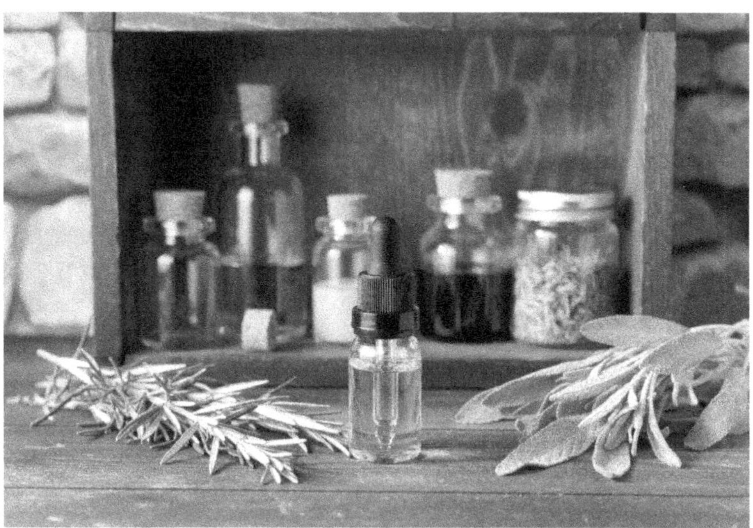

What You'll Need:

- 1 tablespoon of rosemary oil extract
- 1 tablespoon of sage oil extract
- 2 tablespoons of almond oil as a base

Steps to Prepare:

1. Combine the rosemary oil extract, sage oil extract, and almond oil in a clean glass container.
2. Gently shake the container to blend everything together evenly.

Suggested Usage:

Apply a small amount by rubbing it onto your forehead and the back of your neck each day to help enhance concentration and recall.

Important Cautions:

Do not use it if you are expecting a baby or have a history of seizures.

Soothing Greens and Spice Wrap for Ache Relief

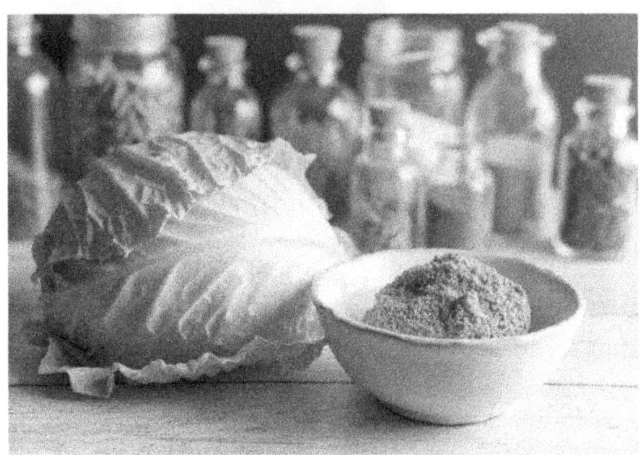

What You'll Need:

- 4 broad cabbage leaves
- 1 tablespoon ground mustard seeds
- 1 tablespoon vegetable oil

Steps to Prepare:

1. Gently heat the cabbage leaves in boiling water for a few minutes until they become flexible.
2. Blend the ground mustard seeds with the vegetable oil to create a smooth mixture.
3. Coat the inner side of each leaf with the mixture, then place them directly on the affected spot.

Suggested Usage:

Apply this wrap to areas with muscle tension or joint discomfort to help ease soreness naturally.

Important Cautions:

Skip this if your skin is easily irritated or if you're allergic to mustard; always test a small area first to check for reactions.

Breath-Supporting Herbal Infusion with Yarrow and Licorice

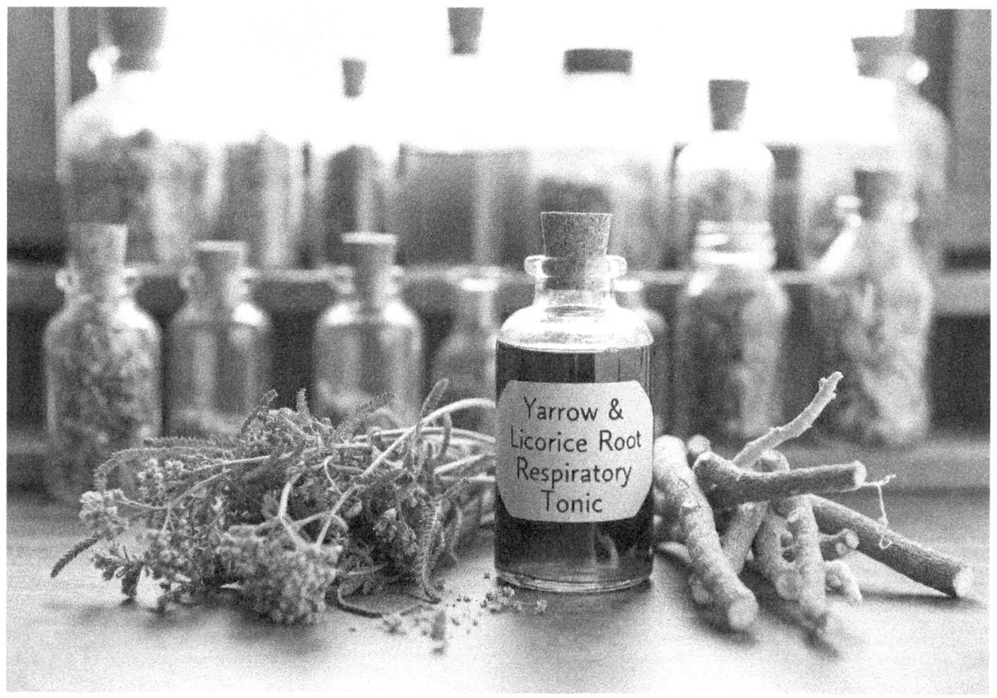

What You'll Need:

- A spoonful of dried yarrow blossoms
- A spoonful of chopped licorice root
- Two cups of clean water

Steps to Prepare:

1. Add the yarrow blossoms and licorice root to a small pot filled with the water.
2. Heat the mixture until it starts bubbling, then lower the flame and let it gently cook for around ten minutes.
3. Take the pot off the stove, pour the liquid through a fine mesh to remove the plant parts, and wait for it to reach a comfortable temperature.

Suggested Usage:

Enjoy one cup of the cooled infusion in the morning and another in the evening to help keep your breathing passages feeling clear and comfortable.

Important Cautions:

Skip this blend if your blood pressure tends to run high, since licorice root might make it worse. Always check with a doctor before trying new herbal mixes, especially if you have health conditions or take medications.

Hawthorn and Ginkgo Infusion for Cardiovascular Support

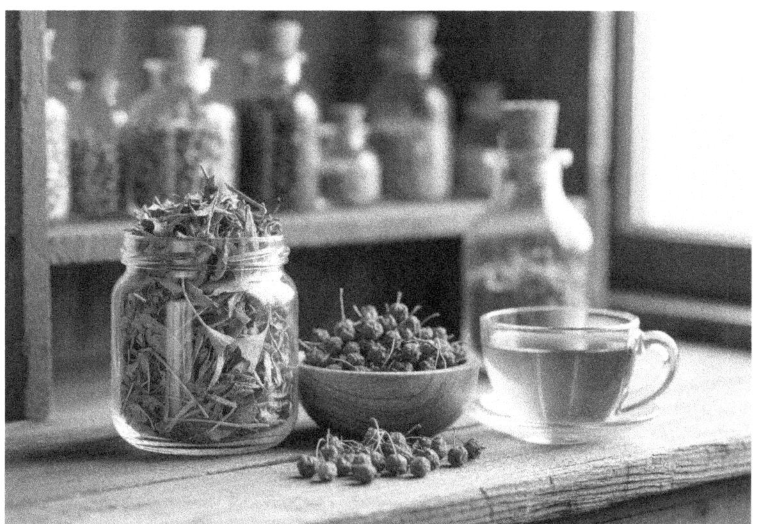

What You'll Need:

- 1 teaspoon of dried ginkgo leaves
- 1 teaspoon of dried hawthorn fruits
- 2 cups of fresh water

Steps to Prepare:

1. Heat the water until it just starts to bubble.
2. Add the ginkgo leaves and hawthorn fruits to the hot water.
3. Let the mixture sit covered for about 15 minutes to draw out the natural goodness.
4. Pour through a fine mesh to remove the plant bits, then enjoy warm.

Suggested Usage:

Have one cup each day to help promote good blood flow and overall heart well-being.

Important Cautions:

Check with your healthcare provider before starting, especially if you're on medicines that thin the blood.

Propolis and Coneflower Vitality Brew

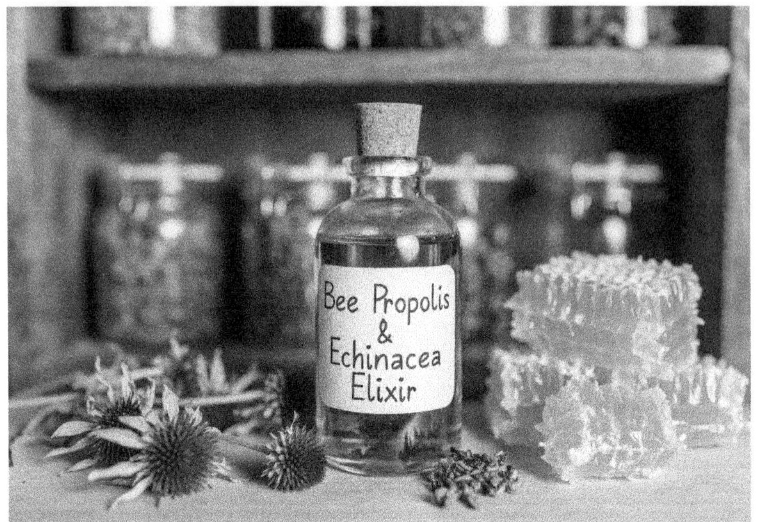

What You'll Need:

- ½ teaspoon propolis extract
- 2 teaspoons dried coneflower (echinacea) herb
- 8 ounces hot water

Steps to Prepare:

1. Pour the hot water over the dried coneflower in a mug.
2. Cover and let it sit for 15 minutes to draw out the goodness.
3. Strain out the herb, then mix in the propolis extract until it blends in.

Suggested Usage:

Sip one serving each morning when sniffles and bugs are common around you.

Important Cautions:

Stay away from this if you're sensitive to bees or their products.

Relaxing Evening Rub

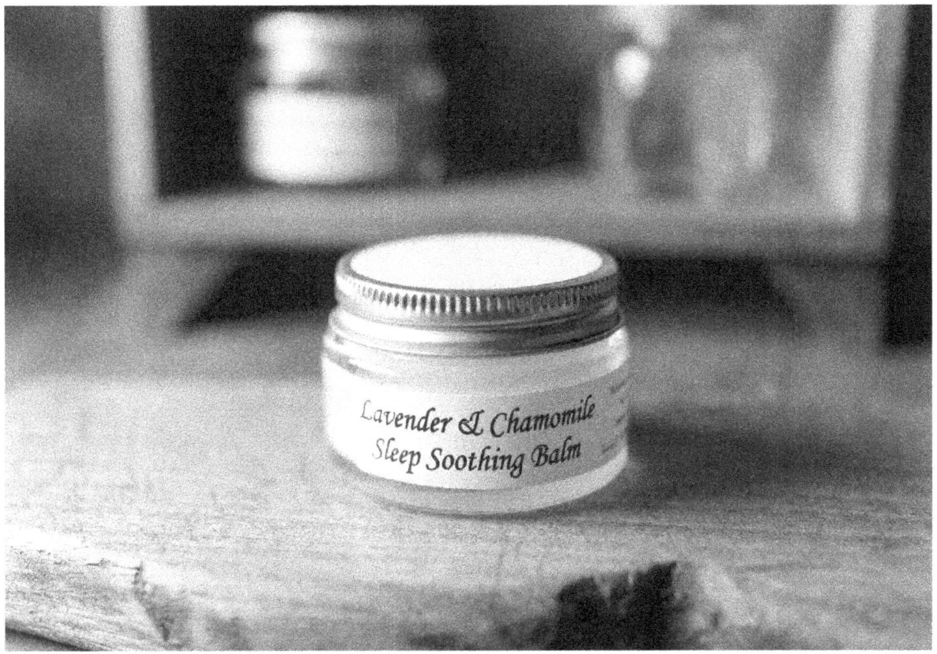

What You'll Need:

- 8 drops lavender essential oil
- 12 drops Roman chamomile essential oil
- 3 tablespoons olive oil

Steps to Prepare:

1. Warm the olive oil gently in a small bowl over low heat until it's just liquid.
2. Stir in the essential oils until everything blends smoothly.
3. Pour into a clean jar and allow it to cool completely before use.

Suggested Usage:

Gently rub a small amount onto your wrists or temples each evening to help unwind and encourage peaceful rest.

Important Cautions:

Keep away from sensitive areas like the eyes; test on a small skin patch first to check for any irritation.

Calming Herb Mix for Everyday Tension

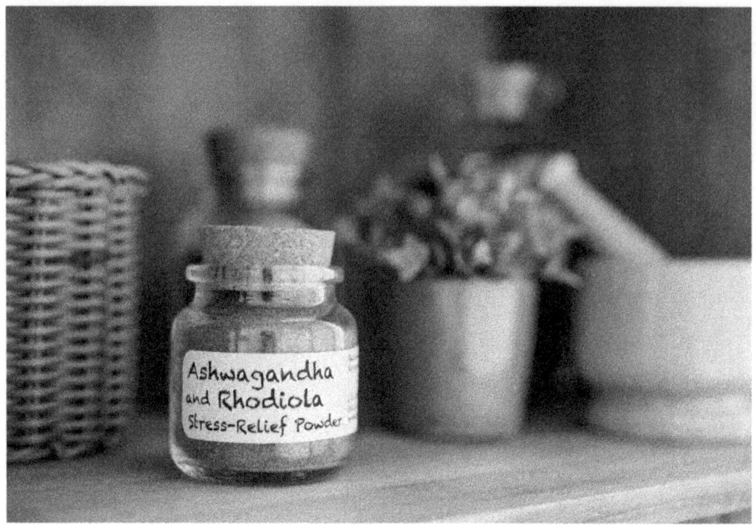

What You'll Need:

- 1 small spoonful of ashwagandha root powder
- 1 small spoonful of rhodiola root powder
- 1 larger spoonful of natural honey

Steps to Prepare:

1. Combine the two herb powders in a small bowl.
2. Stir in the honey until everything blends into a smooth, thick mixture.
3. If you prefer a drink, dissolve the blend in a cup of hot water and stir well.

Suggested Usage:

Spoon up about half a spoonful each day to help ease daily worries and boost your overall vitality. You can eat it straight or add it to a warm beverage for easier intake.

Important Cautions:

Avoid this if you're expecting a baby, as it may not be suitable. Always check with a healthcare provider if you have any health conditions or take medications.

Soothing Wound Care Ointment with Natural Protectors

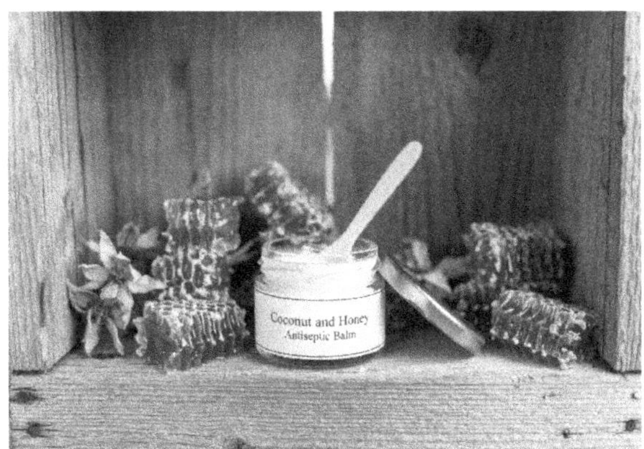

What You'll Need:

- 2 tablespoons of virgin coconut oil
- 1 tablespoon of raw honey
- 1 teaspoon of essential oil from tea tree leaves

Steps to Prepare:

1. Gently warm the coconut oil in a small bowl over low heat until it becomes liquid, if it's solid.
2. Stir in the honey and tea tree essential oil until everything blends into a creamy mixture.
3. Let it cool down, then transfer to a clean jar for storage.

Suggested Usage:

Dab a small amount onto clean minor wounds, scratches, or light burns whenever necessary to help the skin recover naturally.

Important Cautions:

Always test a tiny bit on your inner arm first to check for any skin reaction before full application. Avoid using on deep cuts or if you're allergic to any component.

Evergreen and Spice Cleansing Soak

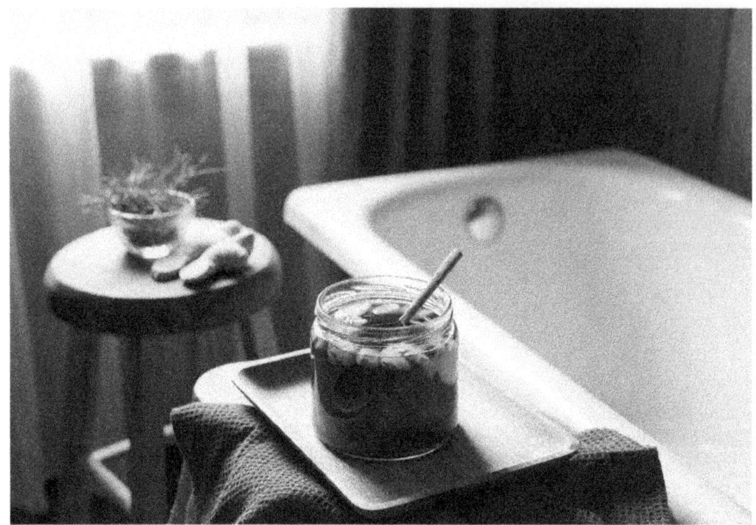

What You'll Need:

- 3/4 cup fresh pine sprigs (or dried if fresh aren't available)
- 2 teaspoons ground ginger
- 3/4 cup bath salts (like magnesium-based ones for relaxation)

Steps to Prepare:

1. Chop the pine sprigs into small pieces and mix them with the ground ginger in a cloth pouch or tied cheesecloth.
2. Secure the pouch to the faucet so hot water flows over it as you fill the tub.
3. Stir in the bath salts once the tub is full, then relax in the water for about 15-25 minutes.

Suggested Usage:

Enjoy this soothing soak once or twice weekly to help refresh and purify your body.

Important Cautions:

Skip this if your skin tends to react easily or if you've had issues with irritation in the past.

Refreshing Herb Spice Purifier Drink

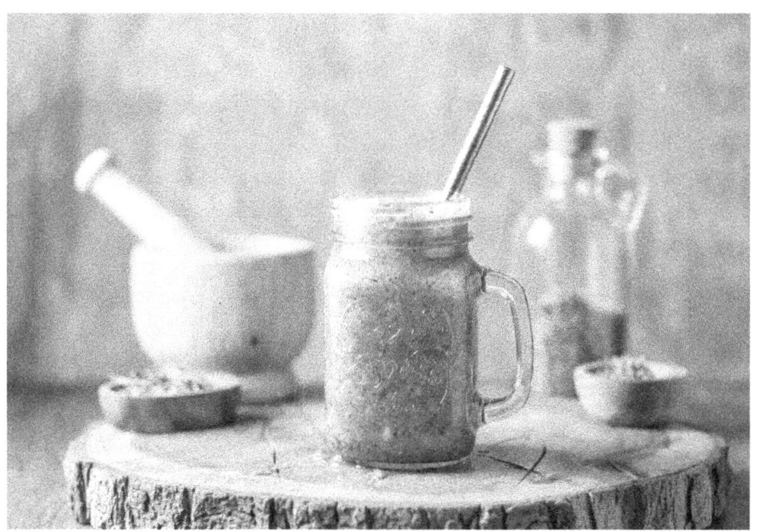

What You'll Need:

A handful of fresh coriander leaves (about ½ cup)
1 teaspoon of ground turmeric
The juice from ½ fresh lemon
½ medium cucumber, roughly chopped
1 cup of coconut water (or light coconut milk for a creamier texture)

Steps to Prepare:

1. Gather everything and add to your mixing machine.
2. Run the machine until the mixture turns velvety and even.
3. Cool it in the fridge briefly before pouring out.

Suggested Usage:

Sip one serving each morning to help flush out unwanted buildup in your system and ease any puffiness or soreness.

Important Cautions:

Skip this if you react badly to coriander or the golden spice.

Rose Hip and Cardamom Soothing Brew for Better Digestion

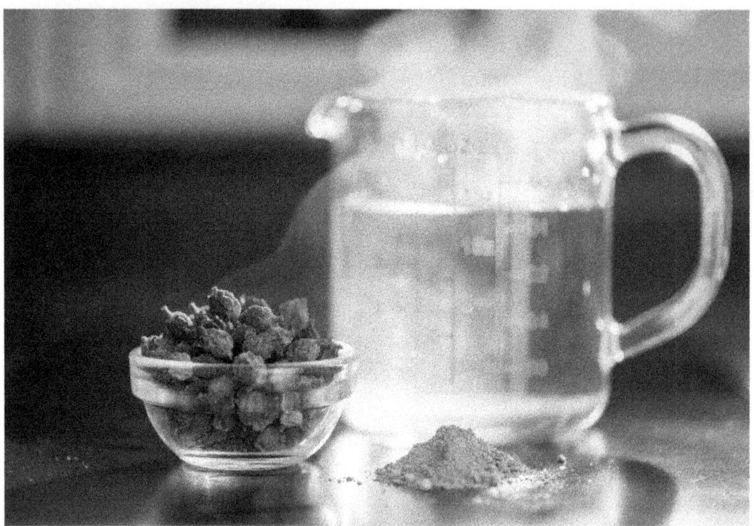

What You'll Need:

- 1 heaping teaspoon of dried rose hip pieces
- A pinch (about 1/4 teaspoon) of powdered cardamom
- 8 ounces of boiling water

Steps to Prepare:

1. Place the rose hip pieces and powdered cardamom into a mug or teapot.
2. Pour the boiling water over them and cover to keep the heat in.
3. Allow the mixture to infuse for 8 to 12 minutes, depending on how strong you like it.
4. Use a fine mesh strainer to remove the solids, then enjoy the warm liquid.

Suggested Usage:

Enjoy one serving right after eating to help ease your stomach and promote smooth digestion.

Important Cautions:

Always check with a healthcare professional before trying this if you deal with any tummy troubles or sensitivities.

Soothing Throat Comfort Blend

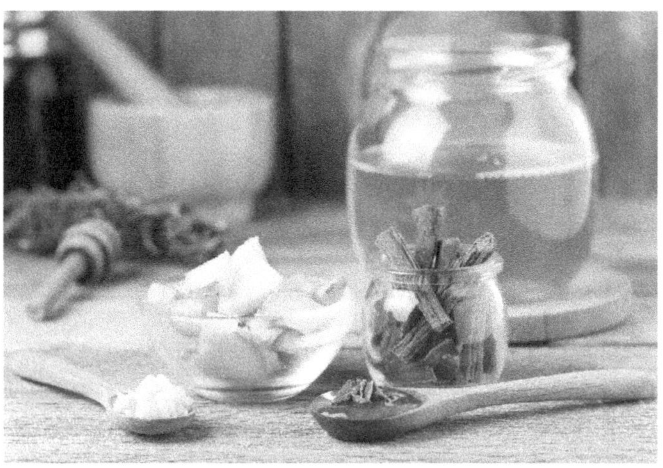

What You'll Need:

- 1 tablespoon grated fresh ginger
- 1 tablespoon dried licorice pieces
- 2 tablespoons raw honey

Steps to Prepare:

1. Add the grated ginger and licorice pieces to a small saucepan with 1 cup of water.
2. Bring to a low boil, then reduce heat and let it gently cook for 10 minutes to draw out the flavors.
3. Take the pan off the heat and pour the mixture through a fine mesh strainer to remove the solids.
4. Once slightly cooled, mix in the honey until fully blended for natural sweetness.

Suggested Usage:

Consume 1 tablespoon every 4 hours or as discomfort arises to help ease throat irritation.

Important Cautions:

Skip this if you deal with elevated blood pressure, as licorice can sometimes affect it.

Berry Boost Defense Drink

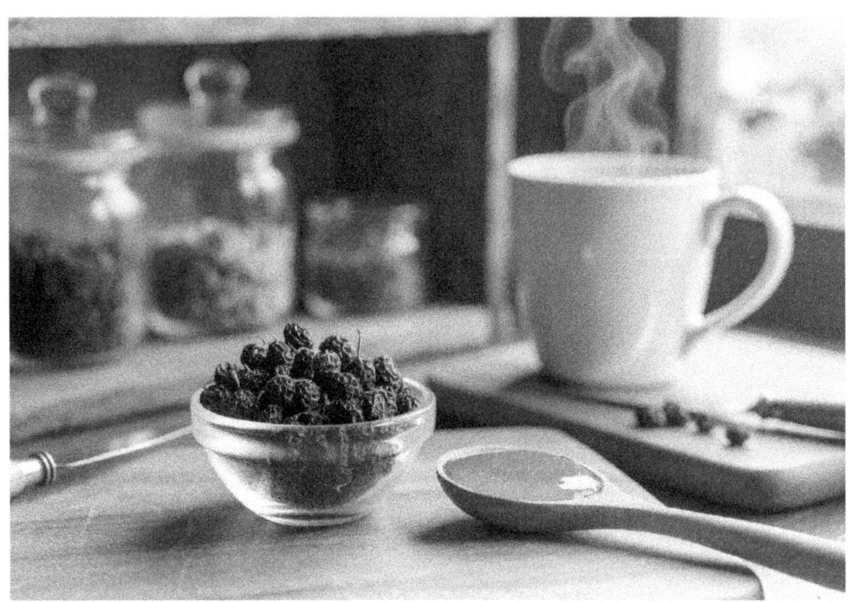

What You'll Need:

- 1 spoonful of dehydrated elder berries
- 1 spoonful of natural sweetener like honey
- 8 ounces of heated water

Steps to Prepare:

1. Let the elder berries soak in the heated water for about 15 minutes to draw out their essence.
2. Filter out the solids and blend in the sweetener until it's fully dissolved.

Suggested Usage:

Sip on one serving each day when sniffles and chills are common in the air.

Important Cautions:

Skip this if you have a known sensitivity to elder berries. Consult a health expert before starting, especially if pregnant or on medications.

Spicy Citrus Vitality Drink

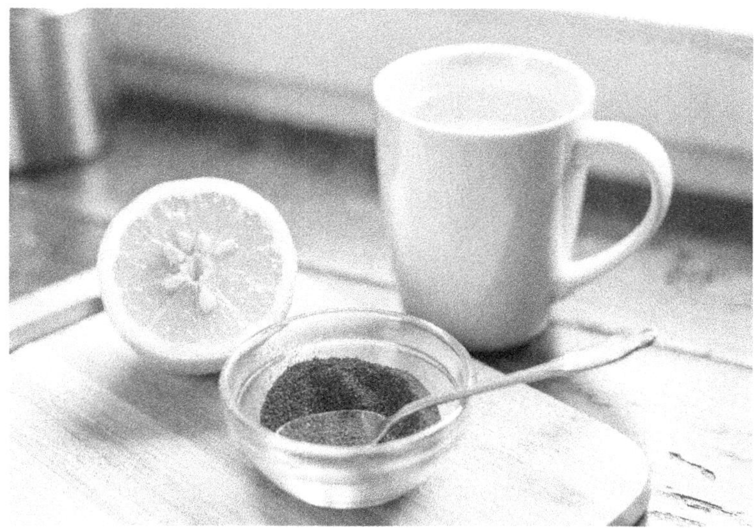

What You'll Need:

- A pinch (about 1/4 teaspoon) of ground red chili pepper
- Fresh squeeze from one whole citrus fruit (like a lemon)
- 8 ounces of comfortably hot water

Steps to Prepare:

1. Pour the hot water into a mug.
2. Add the ground red chili pepper and the citrus squeeze.
3. Give it a good mix with a spoon until everything blends smoothly.

Suggested Usage:

Sip this drink once each day, perhaps in the morning, to encourage better energy and flow throughout your body. For variety, you could try it chilled over ice on warmer days as an alternative twist.

Important Cautions:

Avoid this if you have stomach sensitivities, open sores in the digestive tract, or any ongoing gut discomfort. Always check with a healthcare provider before starting new routines, especially if you take medications.

Relaxing Herb Extract for Peaceful Nights

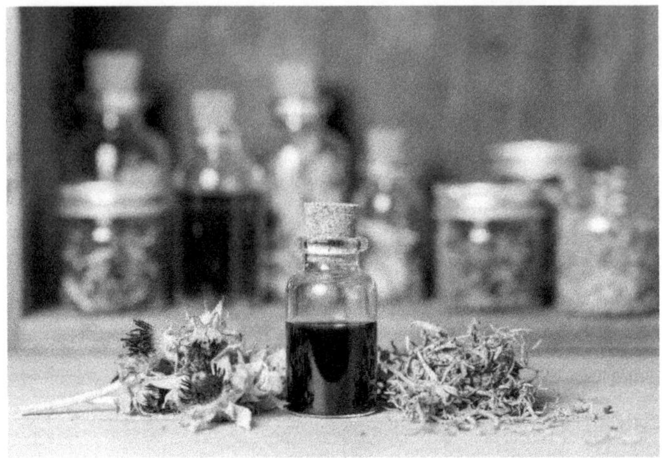

What You'll Need:

- 2 tablespoons of dried passionflower blossoms and vines
- 1 tablespoon of chopped dried valerian rhizome
- 8 ounces of clear spirits like vodka or rum

Steps to Prepare:

1. Add the dried herbs to a clean glass container.
2. Pour in the spirits, making sure the herbs are completely soaked.
3. Secure the lid and keep it in a shady, room-temperature spot for about 4 weeks, giving the container a gentle swirl every couple of days.
4. Once ready, pour through a fine cloth or sieve to remove the plant bits, then store the clear liquid in a small tinted bottle.

Suggested Usage:

Mix 20-30 drops into a bit of water or juice about half an hour before sleep time to help ease into a calm, refreshing rest.

Important Cautions:

Steer clear if you're taking any calming pills or drinking alcohol, as it might make you too sleepy. Check with a doctor first if you're expecting, nursing, or have health conditions.

Energizing Herb Infusion Drink

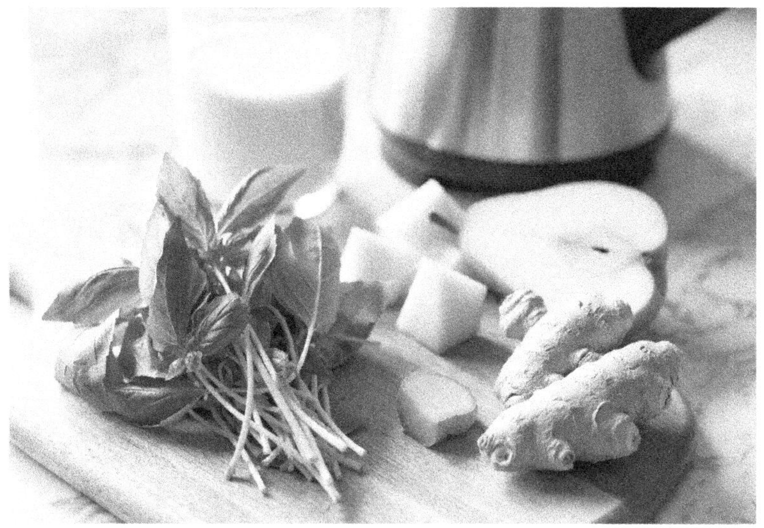

What You'll Need:

- A handful of tender basil sprigs (about 1/3 cup)
- A small piece of peeled ginger (roughly 1/2 inch)
- 1 cup of almond milk
- 1 ripe pear, cored and chopped

Steps to Prepare:

1. Place the basil, ginger, almond milk, and pear into a blender.
2. Mix on high speed until everything combines into a creamy texture.
3. Pour over ice for a cool finish.

Suggested Usage:

Sip this first thing after waking up to kickstart your day with natural vigor.

Important Cautions:

Skip this if you have sensitivities to basil or ginger, and consult a doctor if you're pregnant or on medications.

Soothing Digestive Infusion

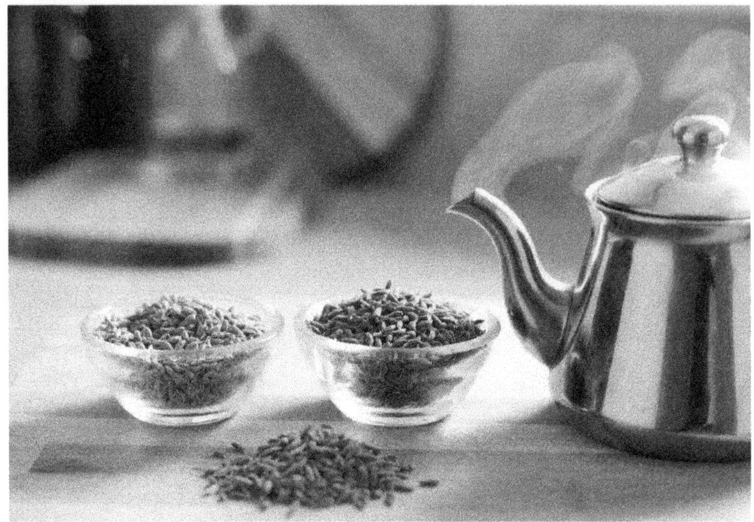

What You'll Need:

- 1 teaspoon whole fennel seeds
- 1/2 teaspoon whole cumin seeds
- 1 cup boiling water

Steps to Prepare:

1. Add the fennel and cumin seeds to a heat-safe cup.
2. Pour in the boiling water and cover to keep the warmth in.
3. Allow the mixture to rest for around 10 minutes so the flavors blend.
4. Pour through a fine mesh to remove the solids, then enjoy the warm drink.

Suggested Usage:

Sip on this brew right after a meal to ease tummy swelling and discomfort from trapped air.

Important Cautions:

Skip this if you know you're sensitive to fennel or cumin seeds. Always check with a doctor if you have ongoing digestive issues.

Herbal Vapor Inhalation for Breathing Ease

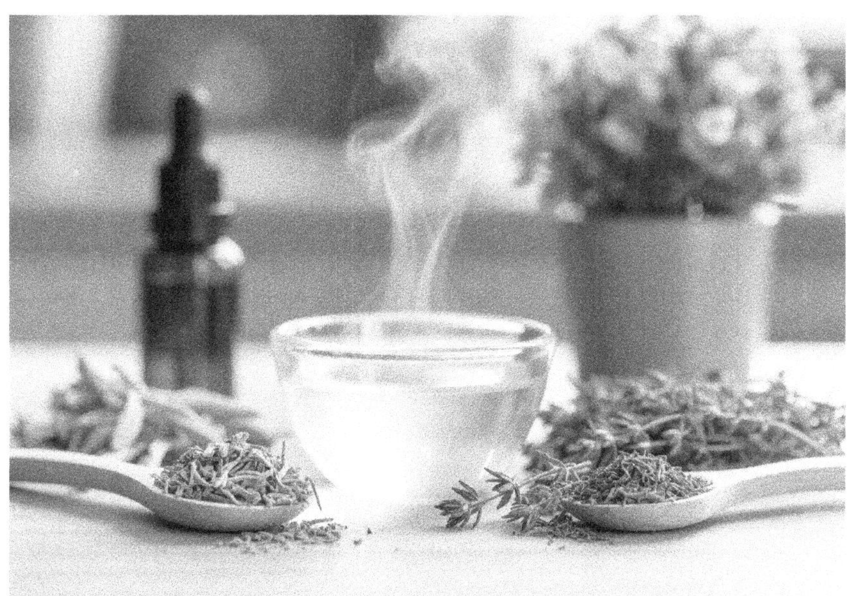

What You'll Need:

- 1 tablespoon dried sage leaves
- 1 tablespoon dried thyme leaves
- A wide bowl of freshly boiled water

Steps to Prepare:

1. Fill a large bowl with boiling water.
2. Stir in the dried sage and thyme, allowing them to release their scents as they float.
3. Lean over the bowl, draping a clean towel over your head to create a tent that holds in the rising vapors.
4. Close your eyes and take slow, deep breaths through your nose for 10 to 15 minutes, or until the water cools.

Suggested Usage:

Try this when you're dealing with blocked sinuses or mild discomfort in your chest from everyday colds. It can help loosen buildup and provide a calming effect on your breathing system. Repeat up to twice a day as needed, ideally in a quiet space for relaxation.

Important Cautions:

Skip this if your lungs are easily irritated or if you have conditions like asthma. Always test for sensitivity by starting with shorter sessions, and stop if you feel any discomfort. Consult a doctor before trying if you have ongoing health issues.

Spicy Garlic Tonic for Stronger Immunity

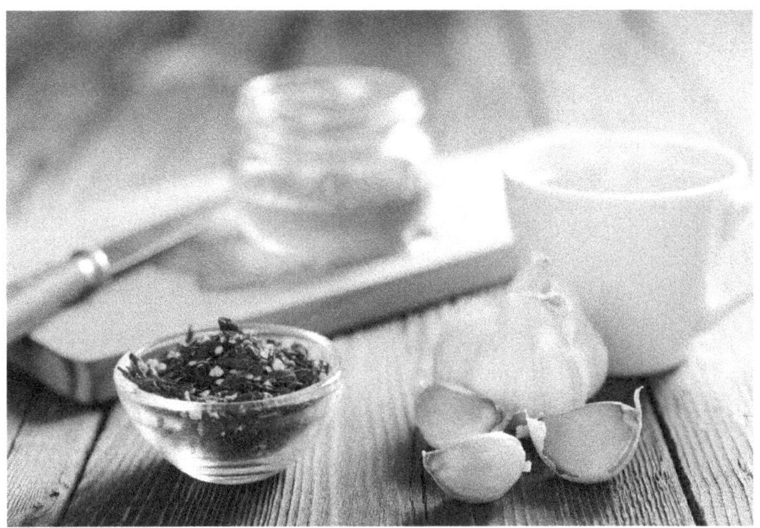

What You'll Need:

- 1 tablespoon red pepper flakes
- 3 garlic cloves, finely chopped
- 1 tablespoon honey
- 1 cup warm water

Steps to Prepare:

1. Add the red pepper flakes and chopped garlic to the warm water.
2. Let it sit for 10 minutes so the flavors can blend.
3. Strain out the solids, then stir in the honey until it dissolves.

Suggested Usage:

Sip one full cup once a day to give your immune system a gentle daily boost.

Important Cautions:

Skip this tonic if you have heartburn, acid reflux, or stomach ulcers—it can be too spicy for sensitive stomachs. Always start with a smaller amount if you're unsure how your body will react.

Soothing Herb Infusion for Tummy Comfort

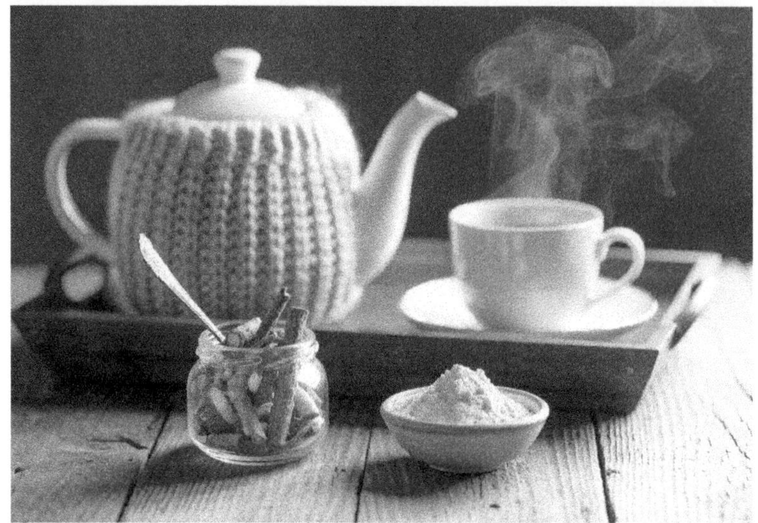

What You'll Need:

- 1 tablespoon dried marshmallow root pieces
- 1 tablespoon slippery elm inner bark powder
- 2 cups boiling water

Steps to Prepare:

1. Combine the root pieces and bark powder in a small pot.
2. Pour in the boiling water and let it simmer gently on low heat for around 10 minutes.
3. Remove from heat, filter through a fine mesh, and sip while warm.

Suggested Usage:

Enjoy one cup each day to help calm stomach upset and encourage smooth digestion.

Important Cautions:

Skip this if you have sensitivities to trees such as birch or elm.

Soothing Herbal Cleansing Soak

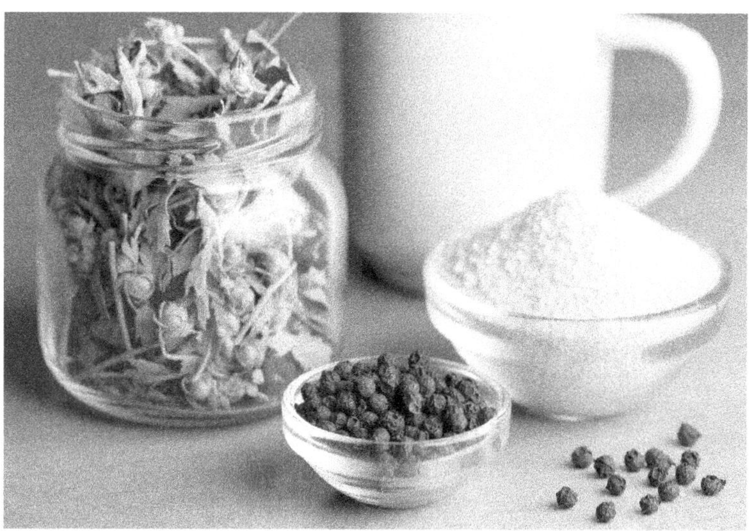

What You'll Need:

- 3/4 cup dried mugwort leaves
- 1/3 cup dried juniper berries
- 1 1/2 cups Epsom salt

Steps to Prepare:

1. Combine the mugwort leaves and juniper berries in a small pot with 4 cups of water.
2. Bring to a gentle boil for 5 minutes, then remove from heat and let steep for another 10 minutes.
3. Strain the liquid into your bathtub as you fill it with warm water, and stir in the Epsom salt until it dissolves.

Suggested Usage:

Ease into the warm water and relax for 25 minutes to help flush out impurities and unwind from daily stress.

Important Cautions:

Skip this if you're pregnant, as some herbs may not be suitable during that time. Always test a small amount on your skin first to check for any irritation.

Nourishing Brew with Hawthorn Fruits and Cinnamon for Cardiac Support

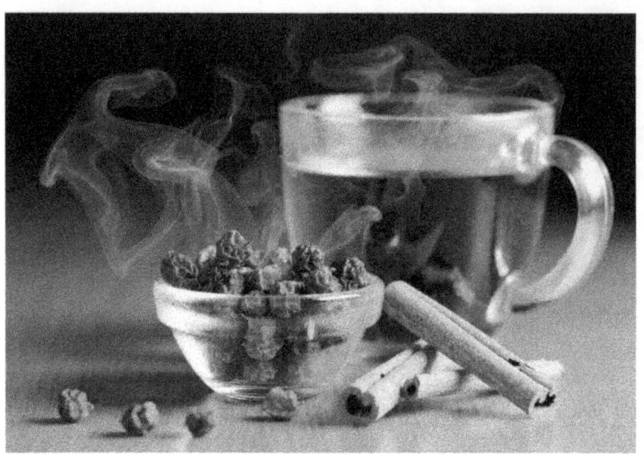

What You'll Need:

- A heaping teaspoon of dried hawthorn fruits
- One piece of cinnamon bark
- Two mugs full of boiling water

Steps to Prepare:

1. Add the hawthorn fruits and cinnamon bark to a small saucepan along with the boiling water.
2. Let the mixture gently simmer on low heat for around 10-12 minutes to draw out the flavors.
3. Pour through a fine mesh to remove the solids, then sip while warm.

Suggested Usage:

Have a single serving each morning or evening as part of your routine to aid in maintaining good blood flow and overall heart vitality.

Important Cautions:

Talk to your healthcare professional first if you take any prescriptions for blood pressure or heart conditions, as this could interact with them.

Peppermint and Thyme Nasal Clearing Vapor

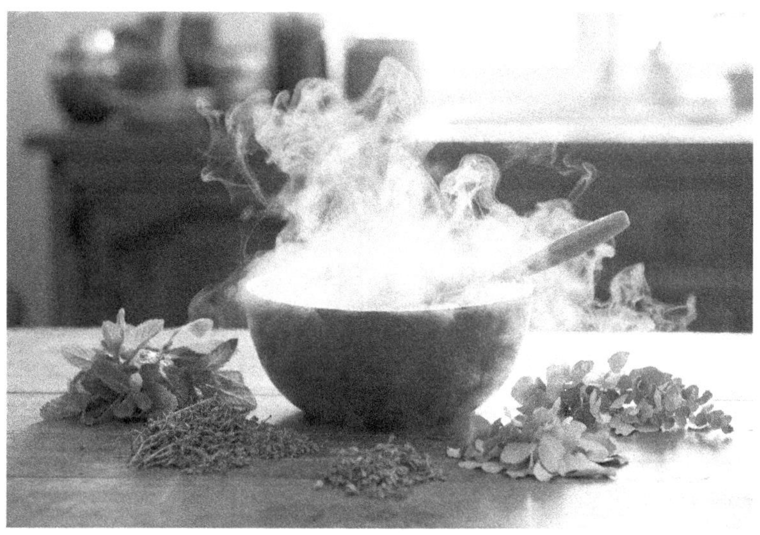

What You'll Need:

- 1 tablespoon dried peppermint leaves
- 1 tablespoon dried thyme
- A large bowl filled with steaming hot water

Steps to Prepare:

1. Place the peppermint and thyme into the bowl of hot water.
2. Lean over the bowl with a towel draped over your head to trap the vapor, and breathe in deeply for about 10 to 15 minutes. This helps open up stuffy nasal passages and ease discomfort from sniffles.

Suggested Usage:

Try this method two to three times daily when you're feeling under the weather from a seasonal bug.

Important Cautions:

Skip this if you're expecting a baby or nursing, as some herbs might not be suitable during those times. Always check with a doctor if you have any health concerns.

Calming Blend Tincture with Yarrow and St. John's Wort

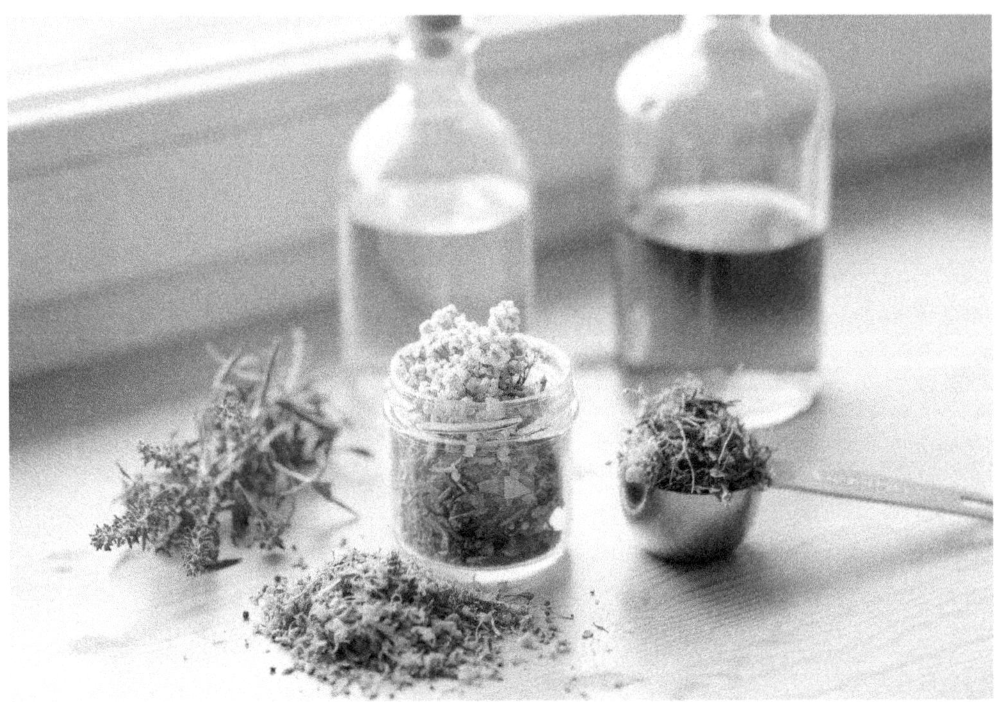

What You'll Need:

- 2 tablespoons of dried yarrow blossoms
- 1 tablespoon of dried St. John's wort leaves and flowers
- 1 cup of high-proof spirit like vodka or rum

Steps to Prepare:

1. Place the dried herbs into a clean glass container.
2. Pour the spirit over the herbs until they're fully covered.
3. Seal the container tightly and store it in a cool, dark spot for about 4 weeks, giving it a gentle shake every few days.
4. After the waiting period, filter out the plant material using a fine mesh or cloth, then transfer the liquid to a dark bottle for storage.

Suggested Usage:

Mix ½ teaspoon into a glass of water or juice once a day to help ease feelings of worry or tension.

Important Cautions:

Do not use it if you're currently on mood-stabilizing drugs or any prescription medicines, as interactions could occur. Consult a healthcare provider before starting, especially if pregnant or nursing.

Soothing Balm for Skin Recovery

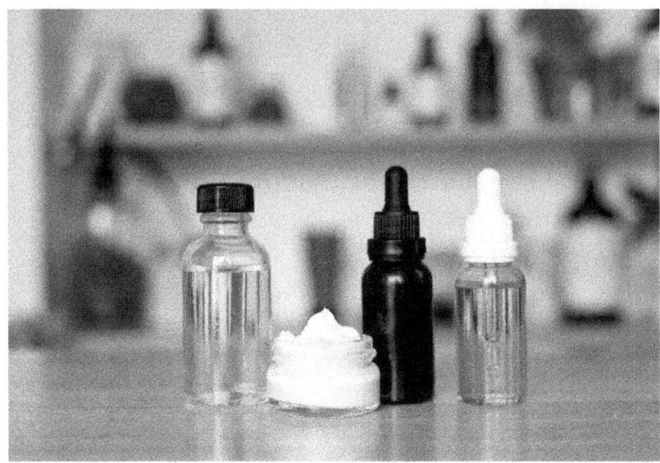

What You'll Need:

- 2 tablespoons of coconut oil
- 1 tablespoon of vitamin E oil
- 5 drops of lavender essential oil

Steps to Prepare:

1. If the coconut oil is solid, gently warm it in a bowl over hot water until it melts.
2. Stir in the vitamin E oil and lavender essential oil until everything blends smoothly.
3. Pour the mixture into a clean container and let it cool to room temperature.

Suggested Usage:

Rub a small amount onto minor scrapes, old marks, or rough patches whenever you notice discomfort or dryness to help nourish and calm the area.

Important Cautions:

Always test a tiny bit on your inner arm first to check for any skin reaction, and wait 24 hours before full use.

Energizing Mint and Citrus Petal Infusion

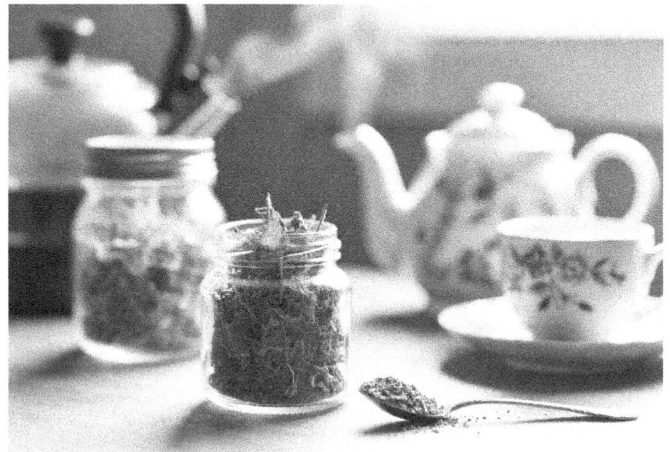

What You'll Need:

- 2 teaspoons of dried mint foliage
- 2 teaspoons of dried citrus flower petals
- 8 ounces of boiling water

Steps to Prepare:

1. Place the mint foliage and citrus flower petals into a heat-safe mug or teapot.
2. Pour the boiling water over the mixture and let it sit covered for about 8 minutes to draw out the flavors.
3. Filter out the solids using a fine mesh strainer, then sip slowly while it's warm.

Suggested Usage:

Enjoy one serving first thing after waking to help brighten your outlook and sharpen focus for the day ahead.

Important Cautions:

Skip this if you have a known sensitivity to mint plants. Always check with a healthcare provider before trying new herbal drinks, especially during pregnancy or if taking medications.

Herbal Infusion for Sharper Thinking with Ginkgo Leaves and Hawthorn Fruits

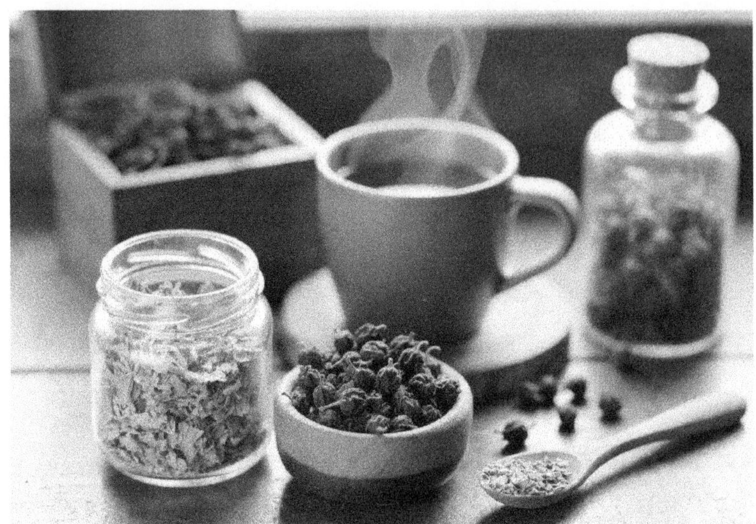

What You'll Need:

- 2 teaspoons of dried ginkgo leaves
- 2 teaspoons of dried hawthorn fruits
- 8 ounces of boiling water

Steps to Prepare:

1. Place the ginkgo leaves and hawthorn fruits into a teapot or mug.
2. Pour the boiling water over them and cover to let the mixture soak for about 10 minutes.
3. Filter out the plant parts and sip while warm.

Suggested Usage:

Enjoy one serving each morning to support better focus and mental sharpness over time.

Important Cautions:

Talk to your healthcare provider before trying this if you're on medicines that affect blood clotting.

Calming Grass and Bloom Serenity Blend

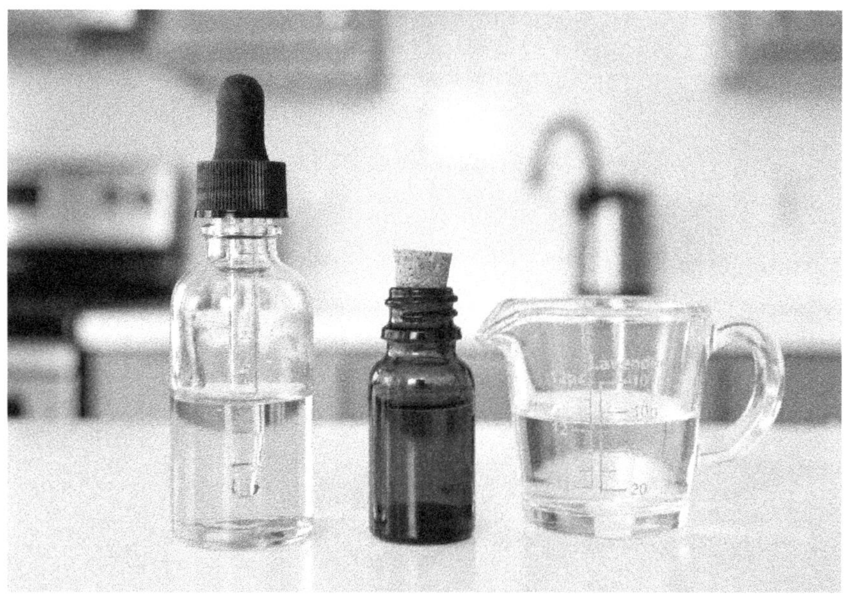

What You'll Need:

- 8 drops lemongrass fragrance oil
- 12 drops lavender fragrance oil
- 2 teaspoons almond oil

Steps to Prepare:

1. Pour the fragrance oils into a clean glass jar along with the almond oil.
2. Gently swirl the jar to blend everything together evenly.

Suggested Usage:

Dab a little on your wrists or neck areas, or add to a room diffuser to help ease tension and promote calm.

Important Cautions:

Skip this if you're expecting or sensitive to lavender scents.

Soothing Blend of Licorice and Marshmallow for Throat Relief

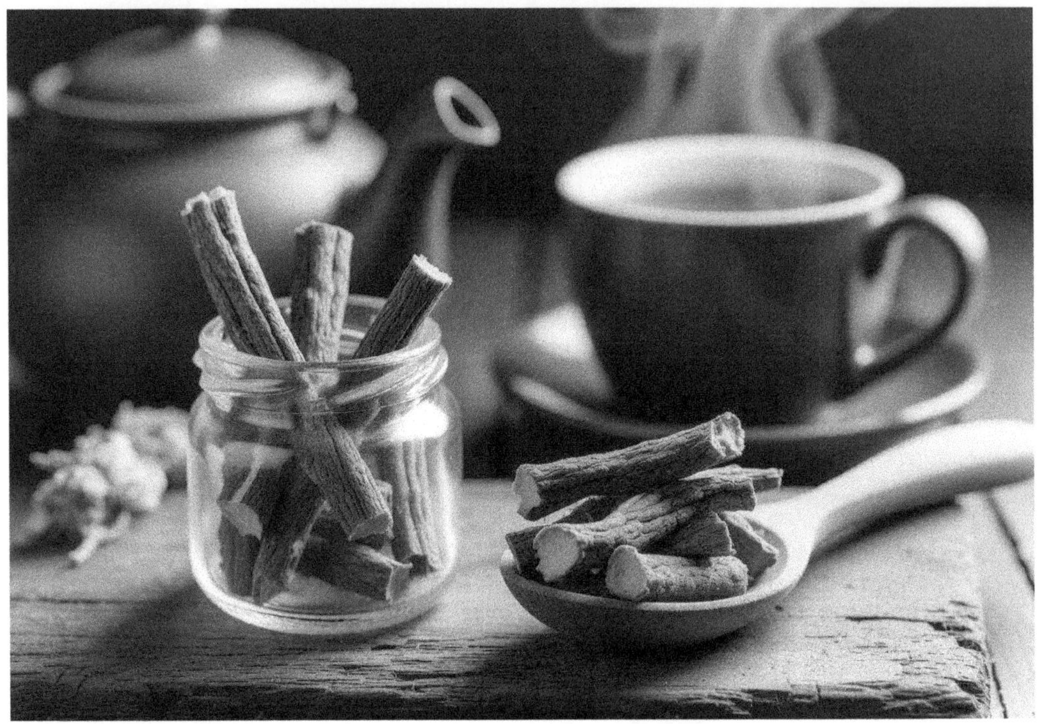

What You'll Need:

- 1 teaspoon of dried licorice root pieces
- 1 teaspoon of dried marshmallow root shreds
- 8 ounces of freshly boiled water

Steps to Prepare:

1. Place the licorice and marshmallow roots in a mug or teapot.
2. Pour the boiling water over them and cover to keep the heat in.
3. Allow the mixture to infuse for about 8-12 minutes to draw out the gentle, coating qualities.
4. Filter out the roots using a fine mesh strainer, then enjoy by taking small, warm sips.

Suggested Usage:

Consume up to two mugs daily when dealing with throat irritation or a dry cough, ideally spaced out to maintain steady comfort throughout the day.

Important Cautions:

Skip this if you deal with elevated blood pressure, as licorice can sometimes affect it. Always check with a doctor if you're pregnant, on medications, or have ongoing health issues.

Nettle and Parsley Cleansing Soak

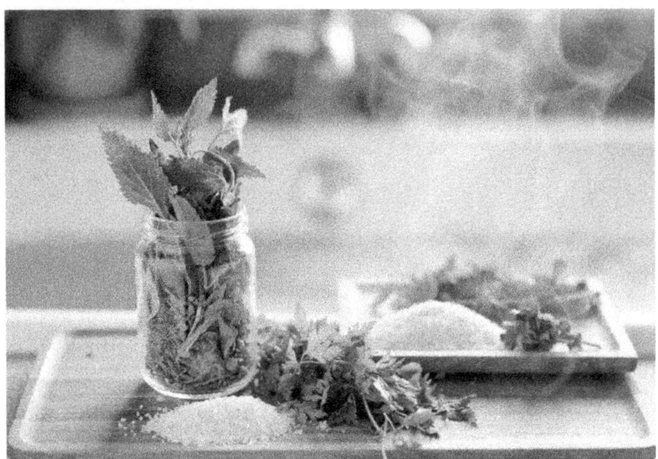

What You'll Need:

- 1 cup of dried nettle leaves
- ½ cup of dried parsley
- 1 cup of Epsom salt

Steps to Prepare:

1. Mix the dried nettle leaves, dried parsley, and Epsom salt together in a bowl.
2. Sprinkle the blend into a tub filled with warm water.
3. Stir gently to help the ingredients dissolve and spread evenly.
4. Get in and relax for 20 to 30 minutes.

Suggested Usage:

This simple soak is great for helping your body release built-up toxins while easing sore or tired muscles. It's a relaxing way to unwind after a long day and feel refreshed.

Important Cautions:

Skip this soak if you have allergies to nettle, parsley, or similar plants in those families. Always check with a doctor before trying new herbal remedies, especially if you have health concerns.

Soothing Cucumber Aloe Blend

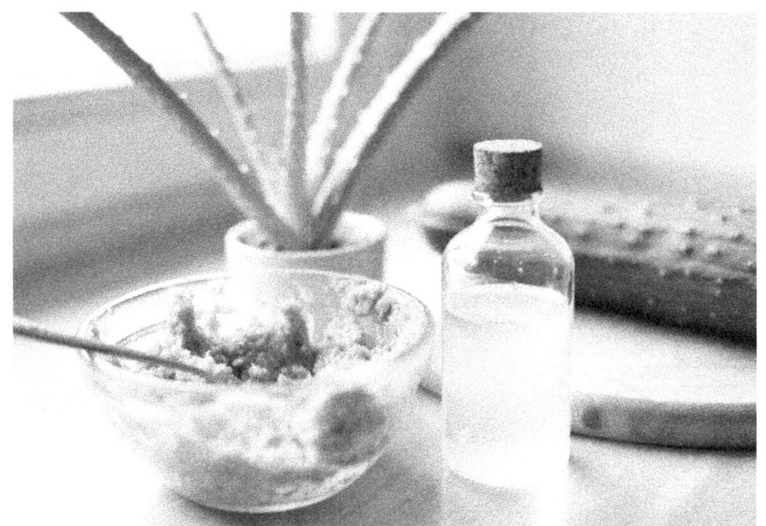

What You'll Need:

- One small cucumber, blended smooth
- Three tablespoons of fresh aloe vera gel

Steps to Prepare:

1. Chop the cucumber into pieces and blend it until it forms a fine paste.
2. Stir the paste together with the aloe gel in a clean container until fully combined.
3. Place the mixture in the refrigerator to keep it fresh.

Suggested Usage:

Spread a good amount onto areas of skin irritated by too much sun to help calm and refresh it.

Important Cautions:

Try a tiny bit on your inner arm first to make sure it doesn't cause any irritation before using more.

Soothing Golden Spice Beverage for Easing Swelling

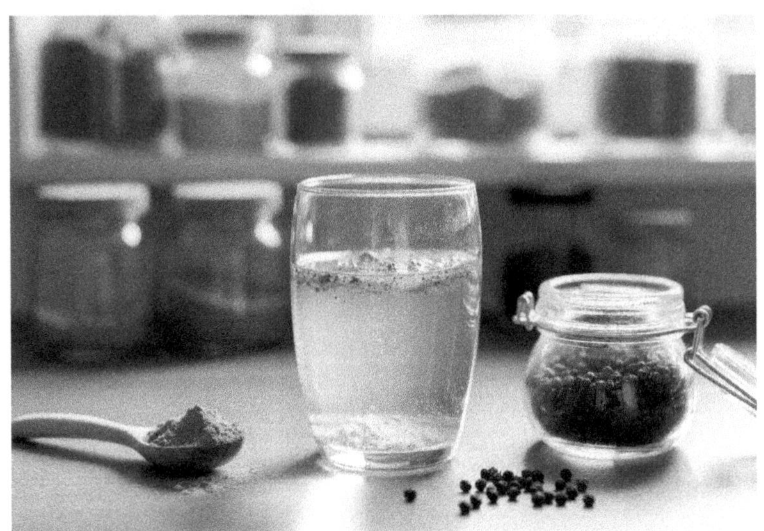

What You'll Need:

- 1 small spoonful of ground turmeric
- A pinch of ground black pepper (about half a spoonful)
- 1 mug of comfortably hot water

Steps to Prepare:

1. Pour the hot water into a mug.
2. Add the ground turmeric and black pepper directly into the water.
3. Use a spoon to mix everything together until it's well blended, then sip it slowly.

Suggested Usage:

Enjoy this beverage once each day to help calm body swelling and soothe achy joints over time.

Important Cautions:

Skip this if you have a known sensitivity to turmeric, and check with a doctor if you're on blood-thinning meds or have stomach issues.

Rosemary and Lavender Scalp Oil for Thicker Hair

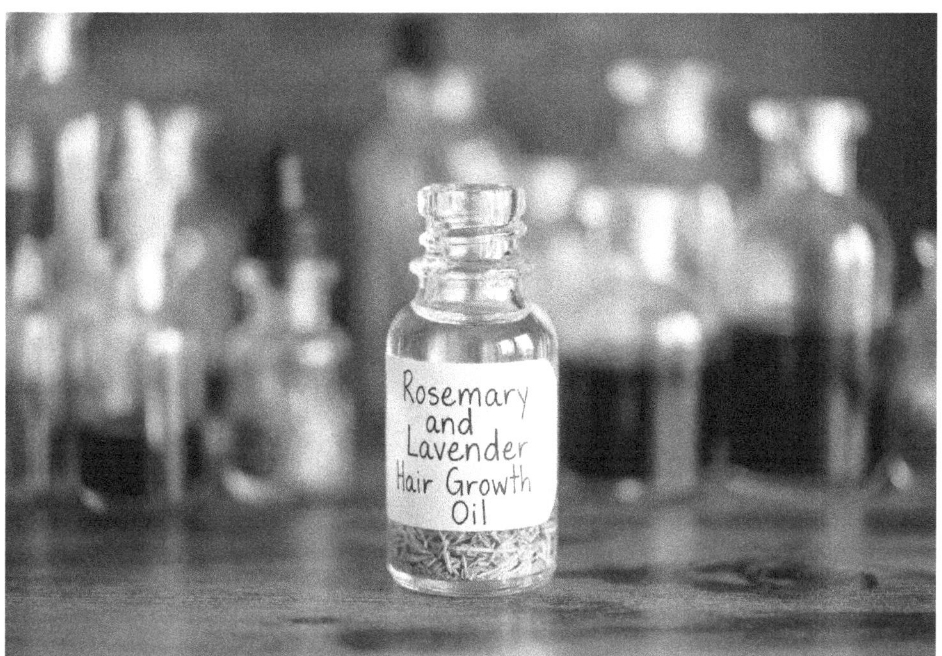

What You'll Need:

- 10 drops of rosemary essential oil
- 10 drops of lavender essential oil
- 1 tablespoon of jojoba oil
- A small clean glass bottle (about 1 ounce size works well)

Steps to Prepare:

1. Pour the jojoba oil into your bottle first.
2. Add the rosemary and lavender essential oils.
3. Put the cap on and gently shake or roll the bottle to mix everything together.

Suggested Usage:

Apply a small amount directly to your scalp 2–3 times per week. Use your fingertips to massage it gently for a few minutes. Leave it on overnight if you like, then wash your hair as usual the next morning. Many people notice softer, stronger hair with regular use over several weeks.

Important Cautions:

Do not use this blend if you are pregnant or breastfeeding. Always do a small patch test on your inner arm first to check for any skin sensitivity. Keep the bottle away from direct sunlight and out of reach of children. If irritation occurs, stop using it and rinse the area with plain oil or mild soap. This is not a substitute for medical advice—consult a doctor for any ongoing scalp or hair concerns.

Refreshing Herbal Vapor for Congested Breathing

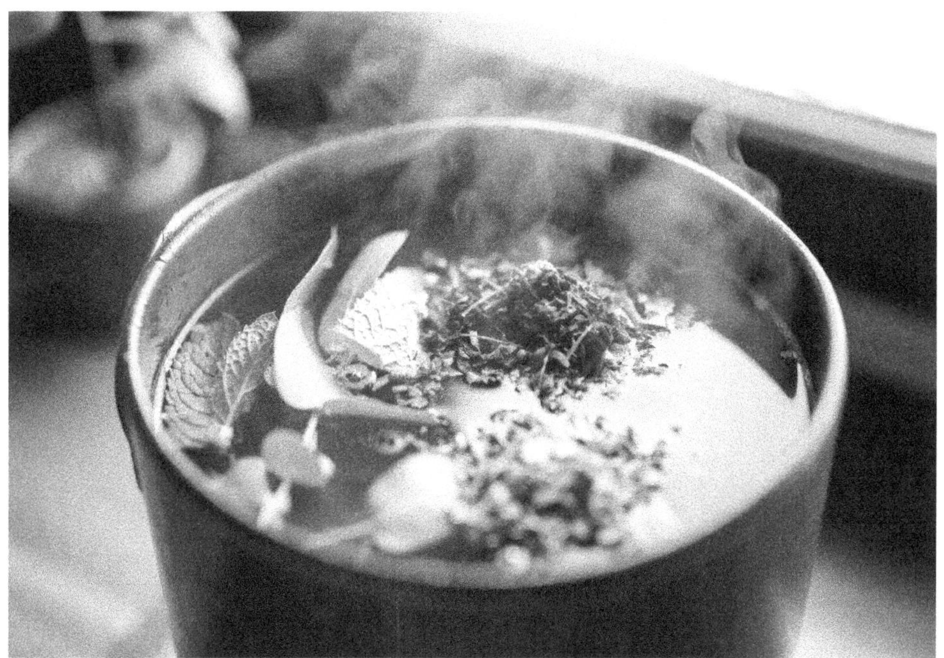

What You'll Need:

- A small handful of crushed mint foliage (about 2 teaspoons)
- A few sprigs of eucalyptus greens (roughly 2 teaspoons, chopped)
- A large container filled with steaming water

Steps to Prepare:

1. Pour the steaming water into your container.
2. Mix in the mint and eucalyptus pieces, allowing them to release their aromas for a couple of minutes.
3. Position your face above the container, using a cloth to create a tent over your head if desired, and breathe in the warm mist slowly.

Suggested Usage:

This method helps open up blocked breathing paths and ease the tightness from stuffy head feelings, ideal during times of discomfort from colds or allergies. Aim for sessions lasting around 8 to 12 minutes, repeating as needed up to twice daily.

Important Cautions:

Skip this if you deal with breathing issues like wheezing conditions or easily irritated lungs. Always test for any personal sensitivities first, and stop if you feel any discomfort.

Fresh Ginger Citrus Reviver

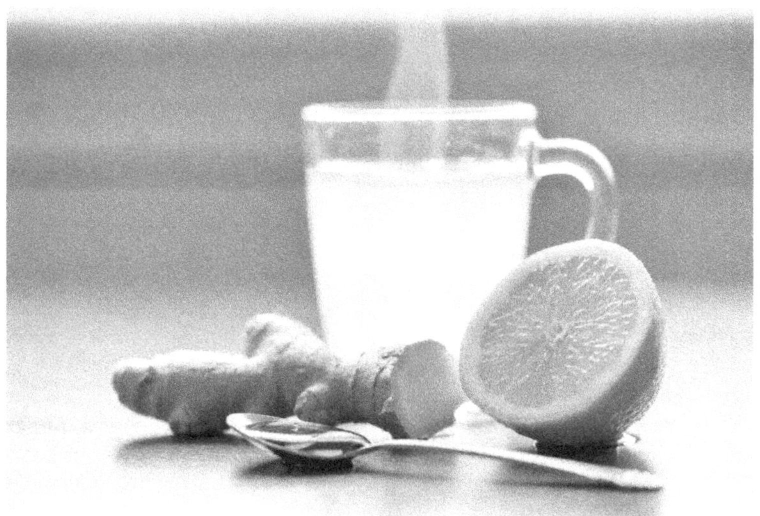

What You'll Need:

- A small piece of fresh ginger (about 2 cm, peeled and sliced)
- Juice from half a fresh lemon
- 1 teaspoon of natural sweetener like maple syrup
- 1 cup of hot water (not boiling)

Steps to Prepare:

1. Place the sliced ginger and lemon juice into a mug.
2. Add the sweetener and pour in the hot water.
3. Let it sit for 5 minutes to allow the flavors to blend, then give it a good stir.

Suggested Usage:

Sip this warm drink first thing each day to help wake up your system and keep your energy steady.

Important Cautions:

Do not use it if you are sensitive to ginger or citrus; check with a healthcare provider if you have stomach issues or are expecting a baby.

Soothing Herbal Blend for Tummy Comfort

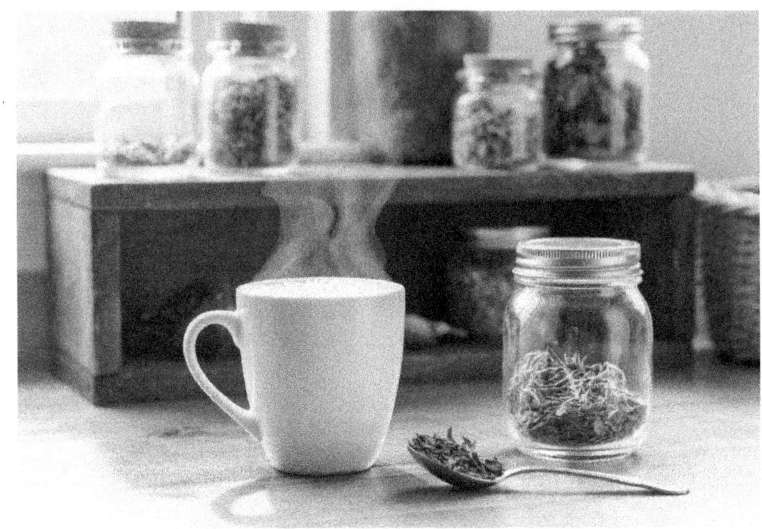

What You'll Need:

- A teaspoon of dried mint leaves
- A teaspoon of dried sage leaves
- One mug of boiling water

Steps to Prepare:

1. Place the mint and sage leaves into a tea infuser or directly in your mug.
2. Pour the boiling water over the herbs and cover the mug to keep the heat in.
3. Let it sit for about 8 to 12 minutes to allow the flavors to release.
4. Remove the herbs or strain the liquid, then sip slowly while warm.

Suggested Usage:

Enjoy a cup following your main meals to help ease bloating and support smooth digestion.

Important Cautions:

Skip this if you're expecting a baby or breastfeeding, as it might not be suitable. Always check with a doctor if you have health conditions or take medications.

Relaxing Bedtime Mist

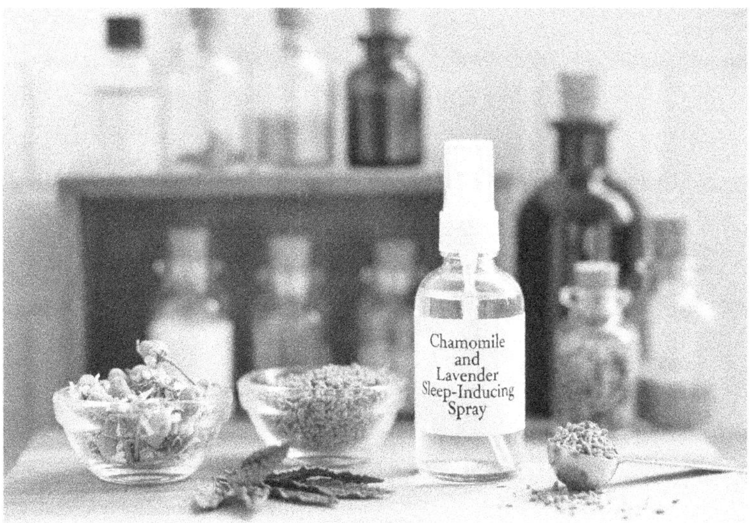

What You'll Need:

- 8 drops of chamomile essential oil
- 12 drops of lavender essential oil
- 1/4 cup purified water
- 1/4 cup witch hazel (helps the oils blend smoothly)

Steps to Prepare:

1. Pour the witch hazel into a clean spray bottle.
2. Drop in the chamomile and lavender oils.
3. Add the purified water to fill the bottle.
4. Secure the lid tightly and give it a good shake to mix everything together.

Suggested Usage:

Lightly spritz your bedding or pajamas about half an hour before turning in for the night to encourage a calm and peaceful rest.

Important Cautions:

Keep away from toddlers younger than 2 years old, as it may be too strong for them. Always do a small skin test first if you have sensitive skin, and avoid direct contact with eyes.

Lemon Thyme Vitality Drink

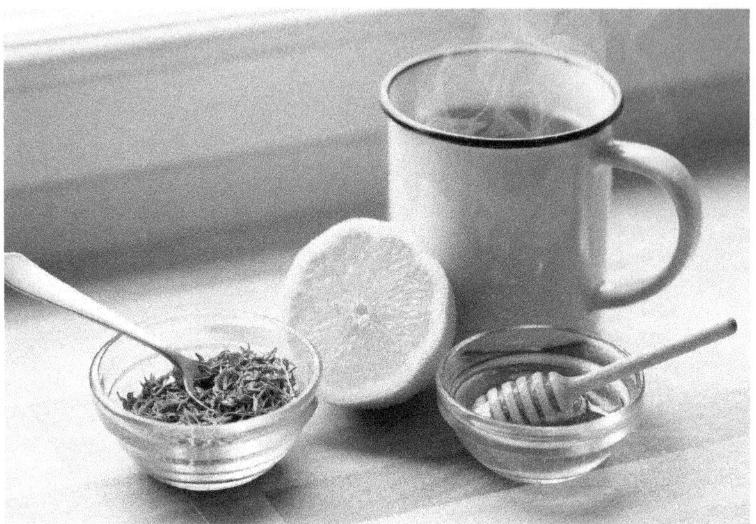

What You'll Need:

- A spoonful of dried thyme leaves (about 1 tablespoon)
- Juice squeezed from half a fresh lemon (roughly 1 tablespoon)
- A small dollop of honey (around 1 teaspoon)
- One mug of boiling water (8 ounces or so)

Steps to Prepare:

1. Pour the boiling water over the thyme leaves in a cup or teapot.
2. Let it sit covered for around 10 minutes to draw out the flavors.
3. Stir in the lemon juice and honey until everything blends smoothly.

Suggested Usage:

Enjoy a warm cup of this drink daily to help support your body's natural defenses and ward off seasonal sniffles.

Important Cautions:

Do not use it if you know you're sensitive or allergic to thyme or similar herbs. Always check with a doctor if you have health concerns or are pregnant.

Soothing Herb Blend for Easing Worry

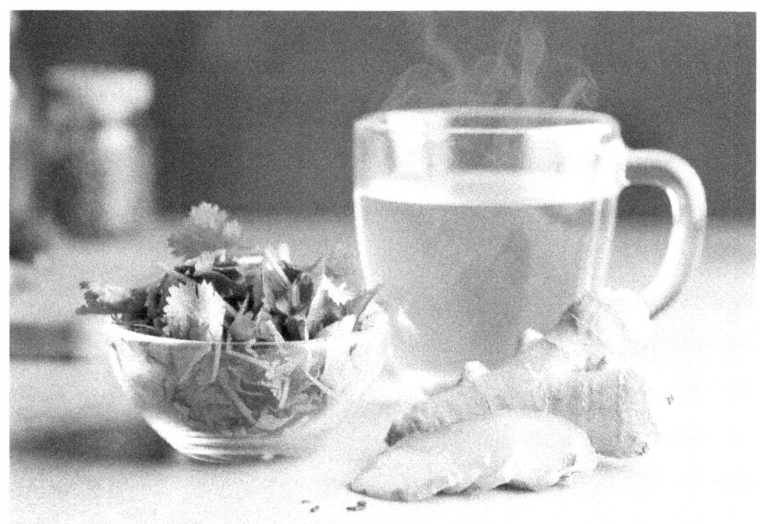

What You'll Need:

- 1 tablespoon of chopped fresh cilantro leaves
- A 1-inch section of fresh ginger, peeled and cut into thin pieces
- 1 cup of boiling water

Steps to Prepare:

1. Add the cilantro leaves and ginger pieces to a heat-safe cup.
2. Cover them with the boiling water and allow the mixture to rest for 10 minutes.
3. Remove the plant parts by pouring through a fine mesh or strainer, then sip slowly.

Suggested Usage:

Enjoy a cup on days filled with tension to promote a sense of calm and relaxation.

Important Cautions:

Skip this if you react poorly to cilantro or ginger, such as with stomach upset or skin irritation.

Soothing Throat Comfort Tea with Elder Blossoms and Honey

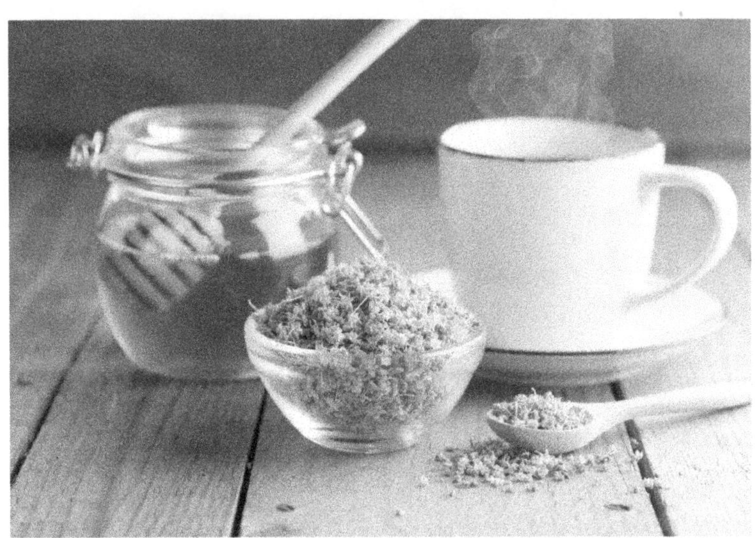

What You'll Need:

- 2 teaspoons of dried elder blossoms
- 1 teaspoon of pure honey
- 8 ounces of heated water

Steps to Prepare:

1. Place the elder blossoms in a mug and pour the heated water over them. Allow them to infuse for 8-12 minutes.
2. Remove the blossoms by pouring through a fine mesh or cloth, then blend in the honey until fully mixed.

Suggested Usage:

Consume this warm drink up to three times each day to help calm throat irritation.

Important Cautions:

Skip this if you know you're sensitive to plants in the elder family. Consult a doctor if symptoms persist or worsen.

Soothing Blend for Respiratory Comfort

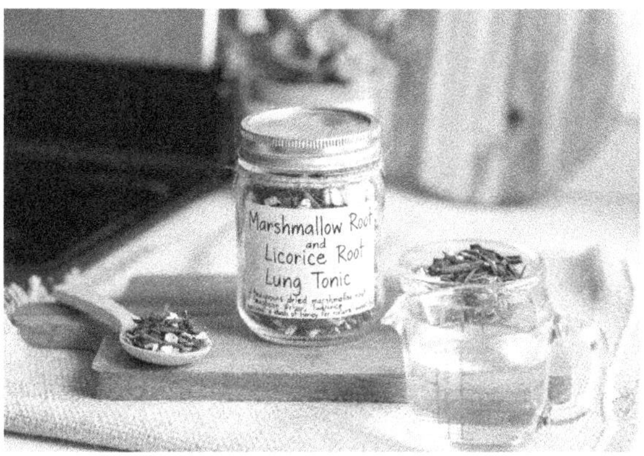

What You'll Need:

- 2 teaspoons of dried marshmallow root
- 1 teaspoon of dried licorice root
- 8 ounces of freshly boiled water
- Optional: A dash of honey for natural sweetness

Steps to Prepare:

1. Place the roots in a small saucepan and pour the boiled water over them.
2. Let the mixture simmer on low heat for about 5 minutes to draw out the beneficial qualities.
3. Remove from the stove, cover, and allow it to sit for another 10 minutes.
4. Pour through a fine mesh strainer into a mug, and stir in honey if desired.

Suggested Usage:

Sip this warm infusion slowly to help ease and nourish your breathing passages, especially during times of dryness or irritation.

Important Cautions:

Skip this if you deal with high blood pressure, as licorice can sometimes affect it. Always check with a doctor before trying new herbal mixes, particularly if you're on medications or have health conditions.

Walnut Shell and Spice Detox Drink

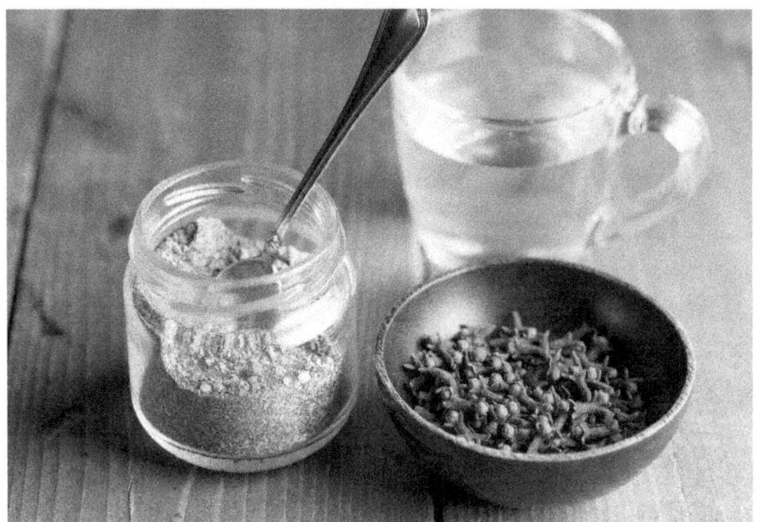

What You'll Need:

- 2 teaspoons powdered walnut hulls from black walnuts
- 1 teaspoon finely crushed clove buds
- 1 cup hot water

Steps to Prepare:

1. Add the powdered walnut hulls and crushed cloves to a mug.
2. Pour in the hot water and let it sit for 5 minutes to infuse.
3. Give it a good stir before drinking.

Suggested Usage:

Sip one mug each morning on an empty stomach to help support your body's natural detox process.

Important Cautions:

Skip this if you're expecting a baby or nursing, and check with a doctor if you have any health conditions.

Ginseng and Cinnamon Calming Brew

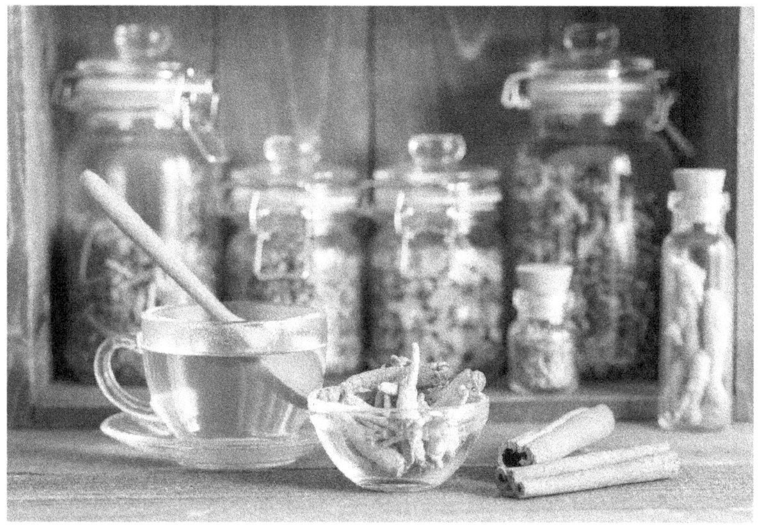

What You'll Need:

- 1 teaspoon of dried ginseng root pieces
- 1 whole cinnamon stick
- 1 cup of boiling water

Steps to Prepare:

1. Place the ginseng root and cinnamon stick into a mug or teapot.
2. Pour the hot water over them and let it sit for about 10 minutes to release the flavors.
3. Remove the solids by pouring through a strainer into your cup.

Suggested Usage:

Enjoy this warm drink when you're feeling tense or need a mental boost. It helps ease everyday worries and sharpens your thinking for better concentration.

Important Cautions:

Skip this if you have high blood pressure, as it might affect it. Always check with a doctor before trying new herbal drinks, especially if you're on medications.

Protective Spice Defense Blend

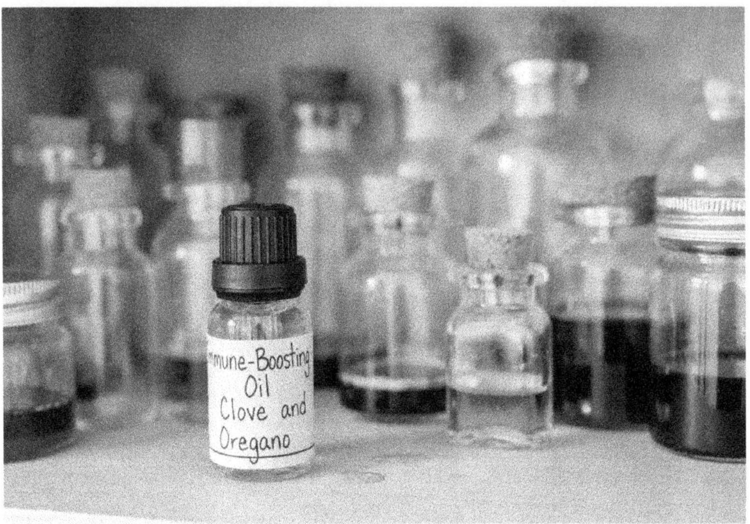

What You'll Need:

- 8 drops clove essential oil
- 8 drops oregano essential oil
- 4 drops lemon essential oil
- 1 tablespoon coconut oil (as a base to dilute)

Steps to Prepare:

1. Pour the coconut oil into a clean glass jar.
2. Add each essential oil one by one.
3. Close the jar and swirl gently to combine everything evenly.

Suggested Usage:

Rub a small amount onto your throat or upper back whenever you want extra defense against everyday bugs. Reapply every few hours if desired.

Important Cautions:

Skip this if you're expecting a baby or have sensitivities to spices like clove, oregano, or citrus. Always do a patch test on your inner arm first to check for any skin reactions.

Calming Herbal Brew for Stress Relief

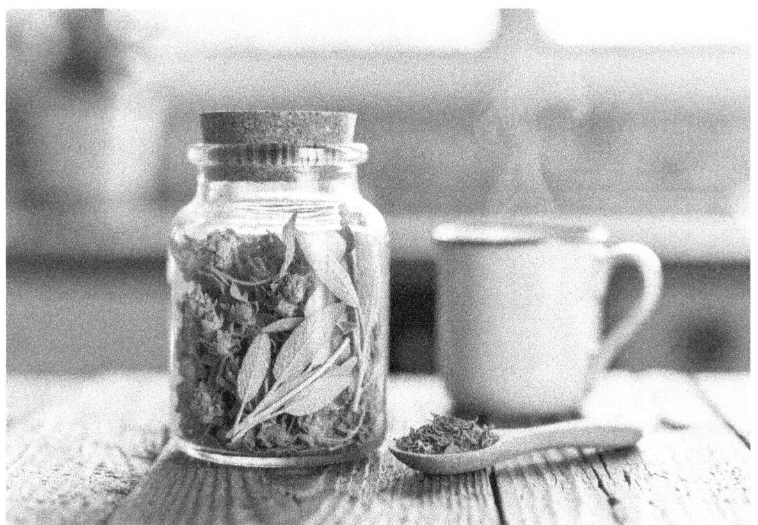

What You'll Need:

- 1 tablespoon dried lemon balm leaves
- 1 tablespoon dried sage leaves
- 1 cup boiling water

Steps to Prepare:

1. Add the lemon balm and sage leaves to a mug or infuser.
2. Pour the boiling water over them and cover to keep the heat in.
3. Allow the mixture to infuse for around 10 minutes.
4. Remove the leaves by straining, then sip slowly.

Suggested Usage:

Enjoy this brew in the late afternoon or before bed to help ease tension and foster a sense of calm.

Important Cautions:

Skip this if you have a known sensitivity to sage or plants in the mint family.

Herbal Blend for Liver Support

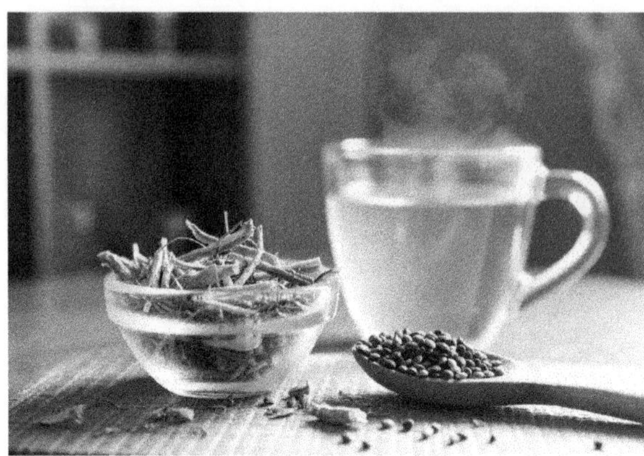

What You'll Need:

- 1 teaspoon of chopped dried dandelion roots
- 1 teaspoon of crushed milk thistle seeds
- 8 ounces of freshly boiled water

Steps to Prepare:

1. Add the dandelion roots and milk thistle seeds to a heat-safe mug or teapot.
2. Pour the boiling water over the mixture and cover it to keep the heat in.
3. Allow it to soak for 15 minutes to draw out the beneficial compounds.
4. Use a fine mesh strainer to remove the plant bits, then let the liquid cool slightly before drinking.

Suggested Usage:

Sip one serving each morning to help your body naturally clear out built-up waste and keep your liver functioning smoothly.

Important Cautions:

Skip this if you react badly to flowers or weeds from the aster group, such as chrysanthemums or marigolds. Always check with a doctor if you're pregnant, nursing, or on medications.

Calming Root and Herb Blend Pills

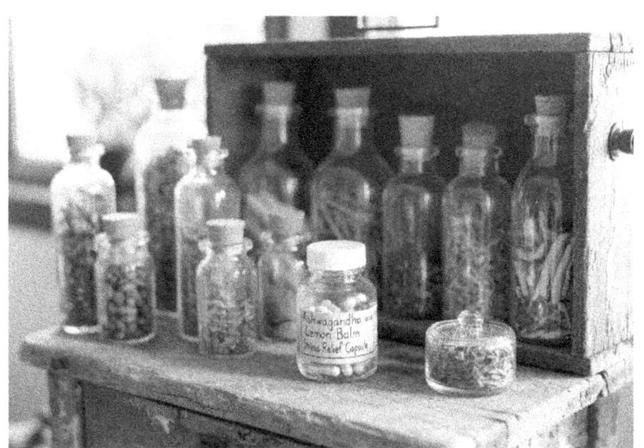

What You'll Need:

- 1 tablespoon of ground ashwagandha root
- 1 tablespoon of dried lemon balm leaves, finely powdered
- Plant-based empty capsules

Steps to Prepare:

1. In a clean bowl, blend the ashwagandha root powder and lemon balm powder until evenly combined.
2. Carefully scoop the blended powder into each capsule half, then press the halves together to seal.

Suggested Usage:

Swallow one filled capsule each morning with water to help manage feelings of worry or unease throughout the day.

Important Cautions:

Do not use this if you are expecting a baby or nursing. Always check with a healthcare provider before starting, especially if you have thyroid issues or take medications.

Herbal Detox Brew for Clean Blood and Liver Vitality

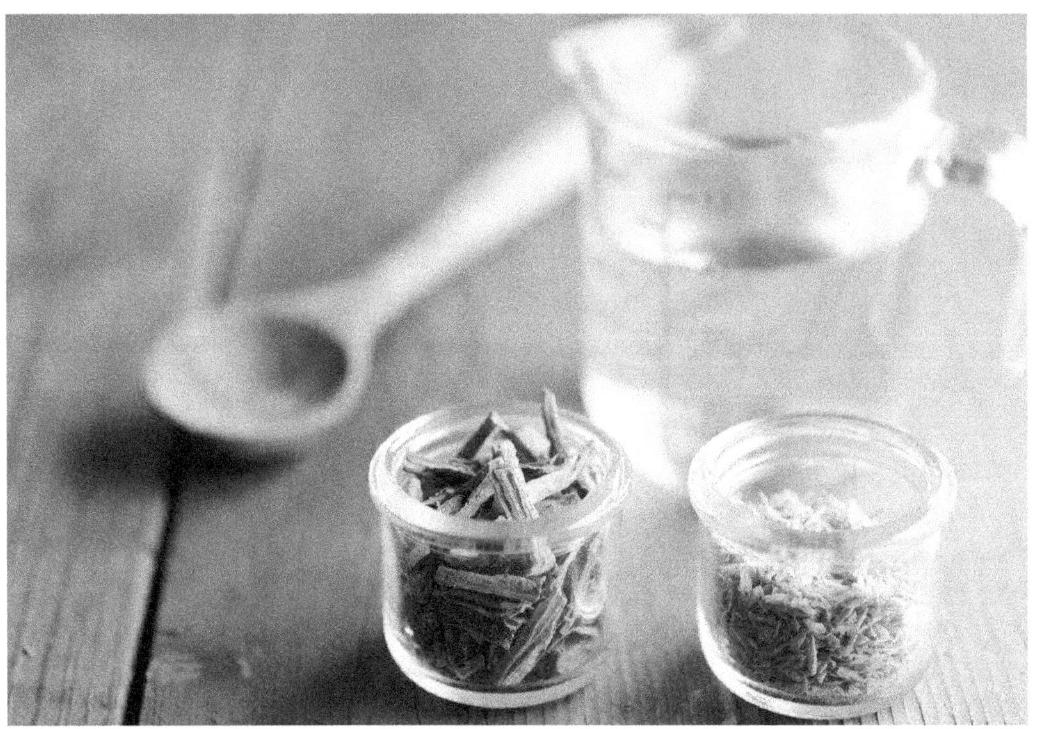

What You'll Need:

- 2 teaspoons of chopped dried burdock root
- 2 teaspoons of chopped dried yellow dock root
- 1.5 cups of fresh water

Steps to Prepare:

1. Add the burdock and yellow dock roots to a small pot with the water.
2. Heat the mixture until it starts to gently boil, then lower the heat and let it simmer softly for about 12 minutes to draw out the helpful compounds.
3. Take it off the heat, cover, and allow it to cool slightly before pouring through a fine mesh strainer into a cup.

Suggested Usage:

Enjoy one cup each day for a span of 5 to 8 days as part of a gentle routine to encourage your body's natural detox process and keep your liver functioning smoothly.

Important Cautions:

Do not use this if you know you react badly to plants like dandelion, as it could cause similar issues. Always check with a doctor if you have ongoing health conditions or take medications.

Soothing Spice Blend for Better Digestion

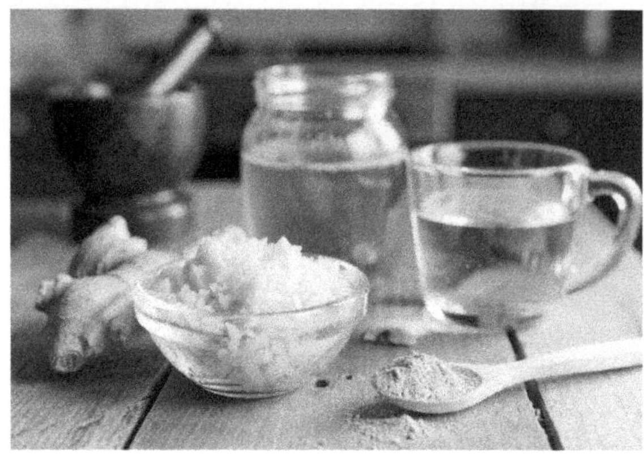

What You'll Need:

- 2 teaspoons finely chopped fresh ginger root
- 1/2 teaspoon powdered cardamom seeds
- 1/3 cup natural honey
- 1/3 cup lukewarm water

Steps to Prepare:

1. Combine the chopped ginger and powdered cardamom in a small bowl with the lukewarm water, stirring gently to blend.
2. Gradually add the honey, mixing until it fully blends into a smooth liquid.
3. Allow the mixture to rest at room temperature for about 45 minutes, then filter out the solids using a fine mesh strainer before pouring into a clean glass container for storage.

Suggested Usage:

Consume a small spoonful right after eating to help ease stomach discomfort and support smooth food processing.

Important Cautions:

Avoid this if you have a known sensitivity to ginger, and consult a doctor if you're expecting a baby or have gallbladder issues, as strong spices might cause irritation.

Calming Blend Extract for Easing Worry

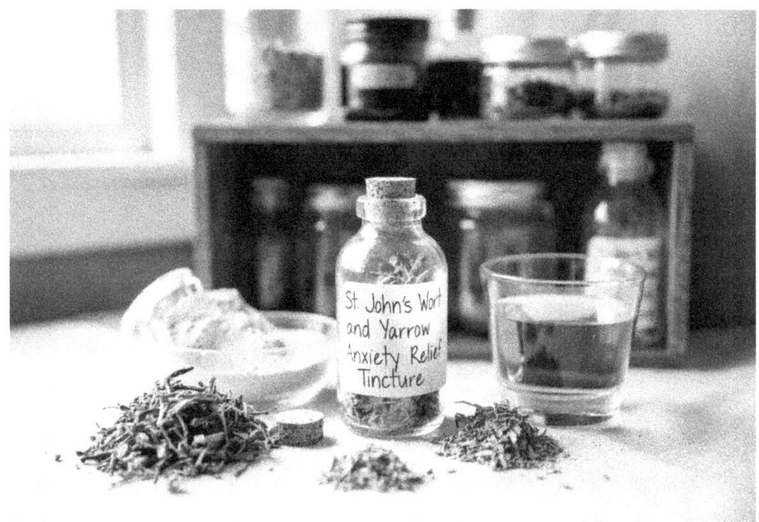

What You'll Need:

- 1 tablespoon of dried St. John's wort herb
- 1 tablespoon of dried lemon balm leaves
- 1/2 cup of high-proof alcohol like vodka or rum

Steps to Prepare:

1. Add the herbs to a clean glass container and cover them completely with the alcohol.
2. Close the container tightly and keep it in a cool, shaded spot for about four weeks, giving it a gentle shake every day or two.
3. Filter out the plant material using a fine mesh or cloth, then transfer the liquid to a small storage bottle.

Suggested Usage:

Mix 20 drops into a glass of water or juice once a day to help soothe nerves and lift your spirits.

Important Cautions:

Steer clear of this if you're on mood-stabilizing medications or expecting a baby.

Boosting Blend for Body Defense

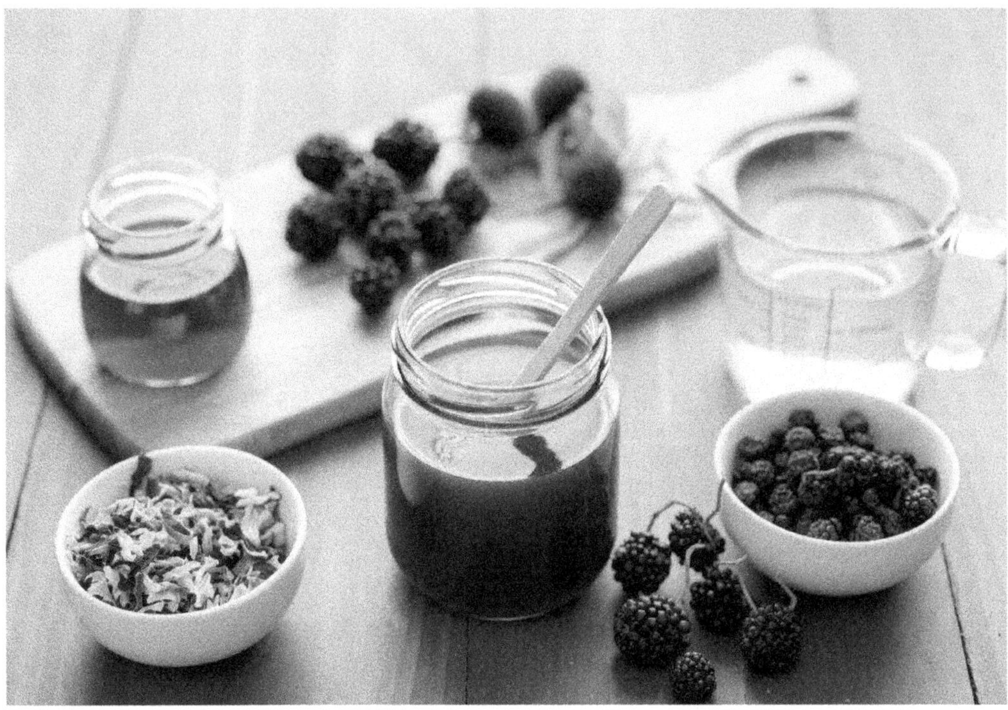

What You'll Need:

- 2 teaspoons of dried coneflower pieces
- 2 teaspoons of dried black elder fruits
- 1.5 cups of fresh water
- 1/3 cup of natural sweetener like bee nectar

Steps to Prepare:

1. Place the coneflower pieces and black elder fruits into a small pot with the water.
2. Heat the mixture gently on low until it simmers lightly for about 10 minutes.
3. Remove from heat, filter out the plant parts, then mix in the sweetener while still warm.
4. Let it cool, then pour into a clean jar and keep it chilled.

Suggested Usage:

Swallow 1 teaspoon two times each day when sniffles or chills are going around.

Important Cautions:

Skip this if your body overreacts to threats on its own, such as in cases where the defense system attacks healthy parts. Always check with a health expert if unsure.

Balancing Herbal Infusion with Clary Sage and Citrus Notes

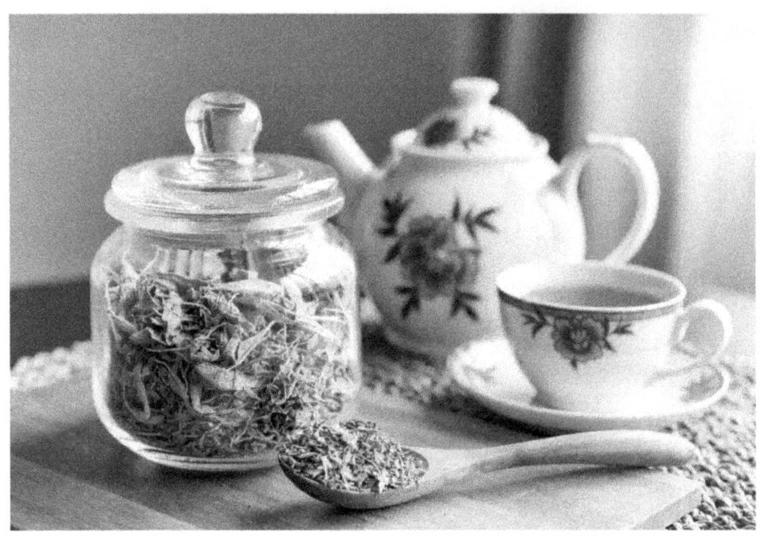

What You'll Need:

- 2 teaspoons of dried clary sage leaves
- 2 teaspoons of dried bergamot herb
- 8 ounces of boiling water

Steps to Prepare:

1. Place the clary sage and bergamot in a tea infuser or small pot.
2. Pour the boiling water over the herbs and cover to keep the warmth in.
3. Let it sit for about 8 minutes to draw out the flavors.
4. Remove the herbs and enjoy the warm drink.

Suggested Usage:

Sip one serving each day to support natural hormone harmony and overall well-being.

Important Cautions:

Do not use it if you are expecting a baby or breastfeeding. Consult a doctor if you have any health concerns before trying this.

Herbal Infusion for Clear Airways

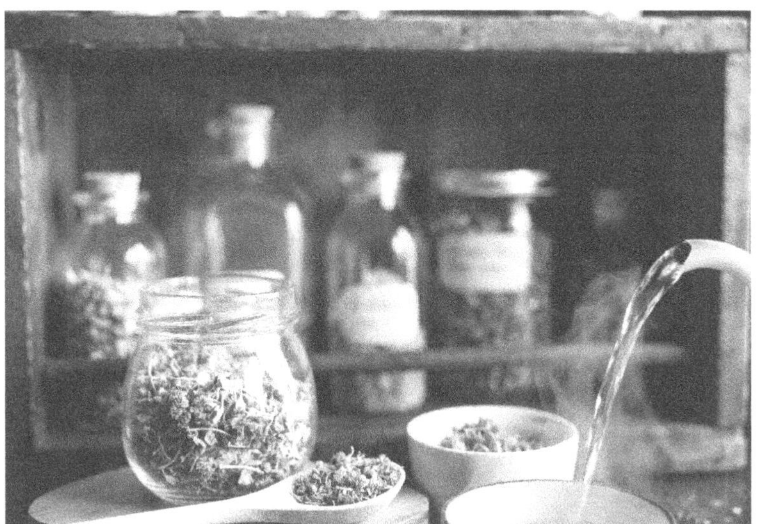

What You'll Need:

- 1 teaspoon dried mullein foliage
- 1 teaspoon dried coltsfoot greens
- 8 ounces boiling water

Steps to Prepare:

1. Add the mullein and coltsfoot to a mug or infuser.
2. Pour the boiling water over the herbs.
3. Cover the container to keep the heat in, and allow it to soak for 8-12 minutes.
4. Remove the herbs by straining, then sip while warm.

Suggested Usage:

Have one serving to help maintain easy breathing and loosen congestion in the chest.

Important Cautions:

Steer clear if you're expecting or facing any liver concerns.

Herbal Infusion for Enhanced Blood Flow

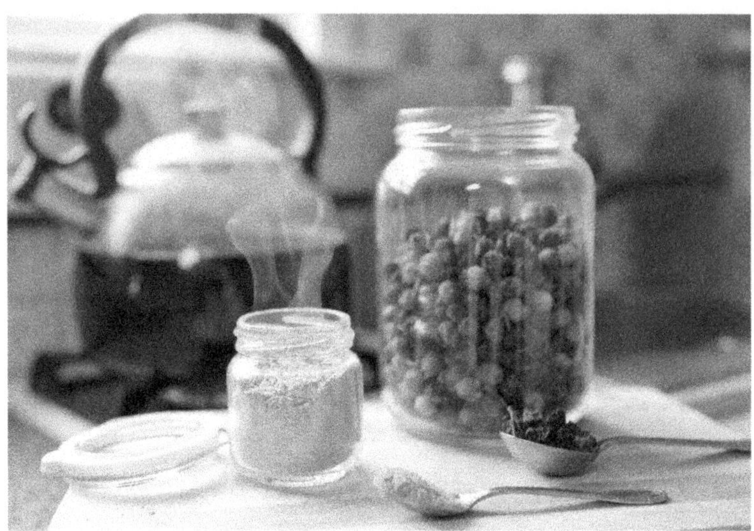

What You'll Need:

- 1 teaspoon of powdered ginseng root
- 1 tablespoon of dried hawthorn fruit
- 1 cup of boiling water

Steps to Prepare:

1. Place the powdered ginseng root and dried hawthorn fruit into a mug.
2. Pour the boiling water over them and let the mixture sit covered for about 10 minutes to draw out the beneficial properties.
3. Filter out the solids and enjoy the warm liquid.

Suggested Usage:

Consume this infusion once a day to support smoother blood movement and overall cardiovascular well-being.

Important Cautions:

Skip this if you're on any prescriptions for heart issues or dealing with a known cardiac problem, as it might interact unexpectedly. Always check with a healthcare provider first.

Soothing Floral Balm for Skin Restoration

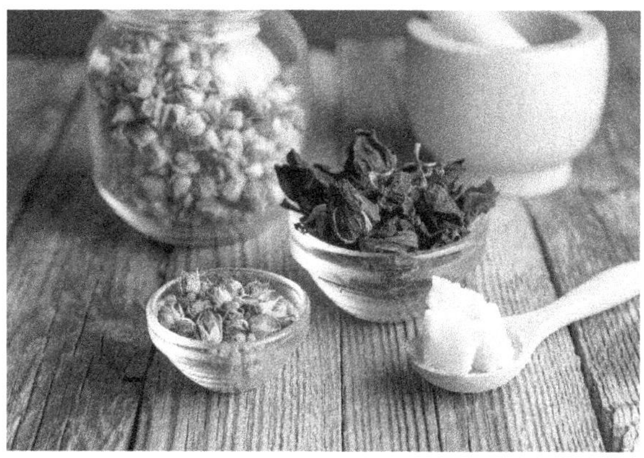

What You'll Need:

- 2 teaspoons crushed dried rose buds
- 2 teaspoons dried hibiscus blooms
- 1/3 cup shea butter

Steps to Prepare:

1. Place the shea butter in a heat-safe bowl over a pot of simmering water to soften it slowly without direct heat.
2. Stir in the rose buds and hibiscus blooms, allowing the mixture to warm gently for about 45 minutes to draw out their gentle properties.
3. Remove from heat, pour through a fine mesh strainer to remove the plant bits, then transfer to a small container and let it firm up at room temperature.

Suggested Usage:

Gently massage a pea-sized amount onto clean, dry skin to help calm irritation and support natural recovery, ideal for everyday moisture in a busy routine.

Important Cautions:

Skip this if you know you're sensitive to rose family plants or hibiscus, as it could cause redness or discomfort. Always test a small patch first.

Soothing Lemon Verbena and Fennel Infusion for Tummy Relief

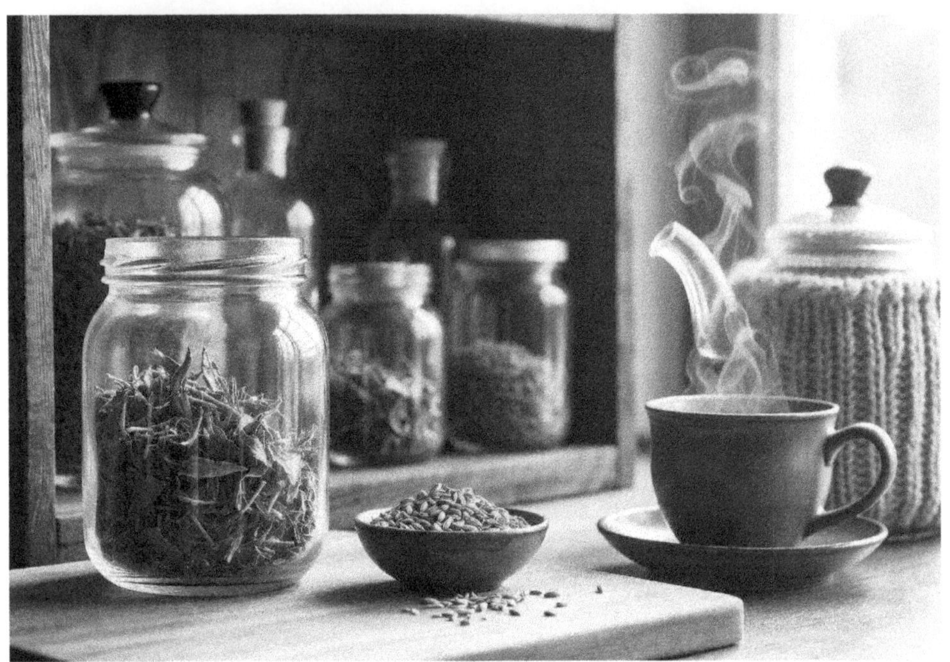

What You'll Need:

- 1 teaspoon dried lemon verbena leaves
- 1 teaspoon fennel seeds
- 8 ounces boiling water

Steps to Prepare:

1. Gently crush the fennel seeds with a spoon to help release their natural oils.
2. Place the crushed seeds and lemon verbena leaves in a tea infuser or directly in a mug.
3. Pour the boiling water over the mixture and cover to keep the heat in.
4. Let it sit for 8 to 12 minutes to draw out the flavors.
5. Remove the infuser or strain out the solids, then sip while warm.

Suggested Usage:

Enjoy a cup following lunch or dinner to support comfortable food processing and ease occasional bloating.

Important Cautions:

Skip this if you're sensitive to fennel or related spices like anise or dill. Check with a healthcare provider if pregnant, nursing, or dealing with ongoing stomach issues.

Spice Blend Defense Oil for Wellness Support

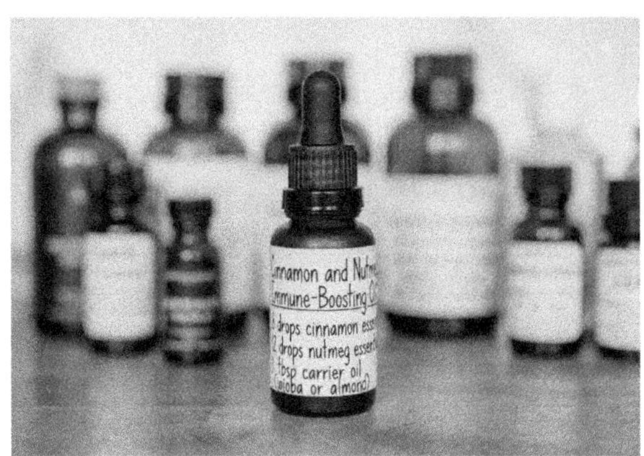

What You'll Need:

- 8 drops of cinnamon essential oil
- 12 drops of nutmeg essential oil
- 1 tablespoon of carrier oil, such as jojoba or almond oil

Steps to Prepare:

1. Pour the carrier oil into a clean, small glass container.
2. Add the drops of cinnamon and nutmeg essential oils.
3. Secure the lid and gently swirl the container to combine everything evenly.
4. Give it a good shake each time before applying.

Suggested Usage:

Rub a small amount onto your upper back or soles of feet to help support your body's natural defenses during sniffle season.

Important Cautions:

Do not use it if you have sensitivities to spices like cinnamon or nutmeg. Test on a small skin patch first to check for any irritation. Keep away from eyes and sensitive areas. Consult a doctor if pregnant or nursing.

Dandelion and Ginger Soothing Brew

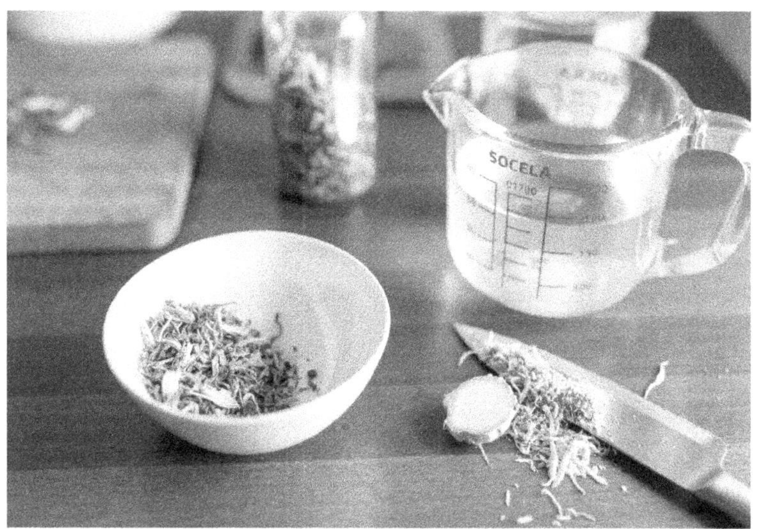

What You'll Need:

- 2 teaspoons of chopped dried dandelion root
- A small piece of fresh ginger, about the size of a thumbnail, finely shredded
- 8 ounces of boiling water

Steps to Prepare:

1. Place the dandelion root and shredded ginger into a mug or teapot.
2. Pour the boiling water over them and cover to keep the heat in.
3. Let it sit for about 12 minutes to draw out the flavors.
4. Pour through a fine mesh strainer into your cup and sip while warm.

Suggested Usage:

Enjoy a cup when your tummy feels off-balance, like after a heavy meal, to help ease discomfort.

Important Cautions:

Skip this if you've been diagnosed with gallbladder issues, as it might not agree with you. Always check with a healthcare provider if you're unsure or have ongoing health concerns.

Calming Capsules with Lemon Balm and Chamomile

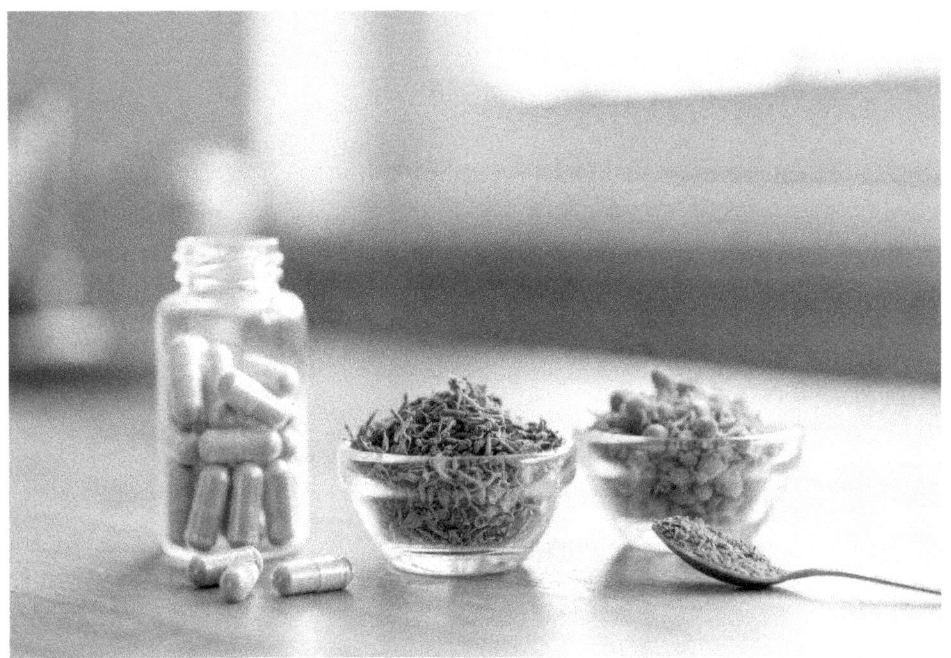

What You'll Need:

- 1 teaspoon dried lemon balm leaves
- 1 teaspoon dried chamomile flowers
- Empty vegetable capsules

Steps to Prepare:

1. Lightly crush the dried lemon balm and chamomile together using a mortar and pestle or your fingers to blend the herbs evenly and make them easier to pack.
2. Mix the two herbs thoroughly in a small bowl until well combined.
3. Carefully open each empty capsule and fill the halves with the herb mixture, packing gently but firmly. Close the capsules securely.

Suggested Usage:

Take 1–2 capsules about 30–60 minutes before bedtime to help calm the mind and encourage relaxation.

Important Cautions:

Do not use it if you have known allergies to plants in the aster family (such as ragweed, daisies, or marigolds), as chamomile may trigger reactions in sensitive individuals. Always start with a small dose to test for personal tolerance. Consult a healthcare provider before use if pregnant, breastfeeding, or taking medications.

Herbal Infusion for Thicker, Stronger Strands

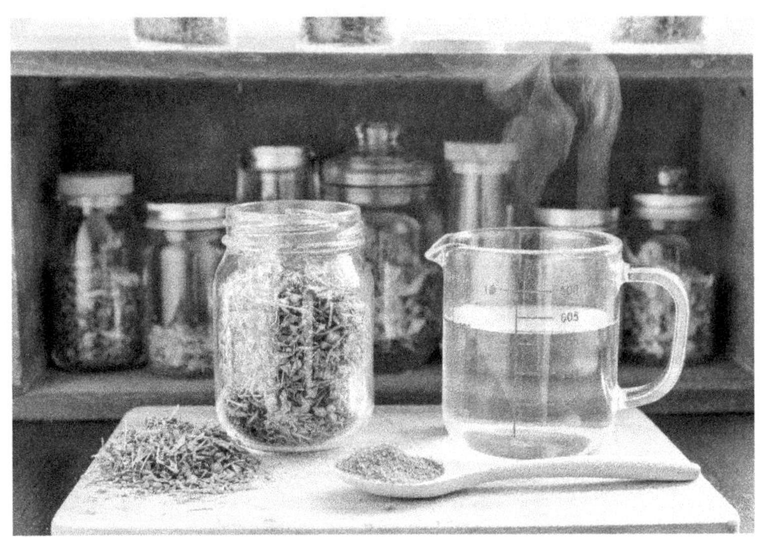

What You'll Need:

- 1 tablespoon of dried horsetail herb
- 1 tablespoon of dried stinging nettle foliage
- 1 cup of boiling water

Steps to Prepare:

1. Add the herbs to a mug or teapot.
2. Pour in the boiling water and cover to keep the heat inside.
3. Allow the mixture to soak for 10 minutes.
4. Pour through a strainer to remove the plant bits, then sip while warm.

Suggested Usage:

Sip one cup every day to support healthier hair development and added resilience.

Important Cautions:

Skip this if you're pregnant or breastfeeding.

Soothing Drumstick Leaf and Spice Drink for Calming Body Aches

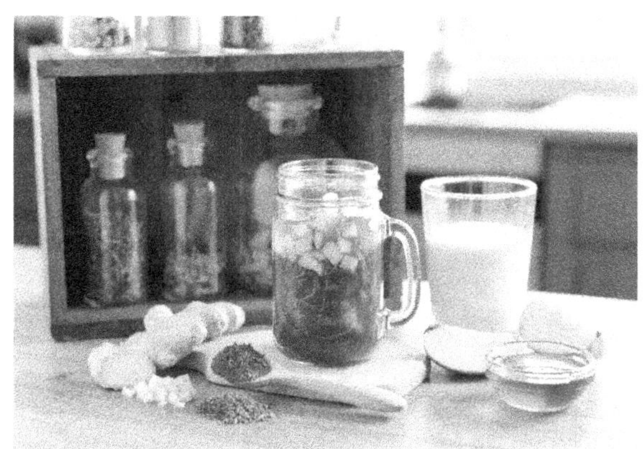

What You'll Need:

- 1 small spoonful of dried moringa leaf powder
- 1 small spoonful of peeled and finely chopped ginger root
- 1/2 cup almond milk
- 1/2 small apple, cored and sliced
- 1 small spoonful of maple syrup

Steps to Prepare:

1. Add the moringa powder, chopped ginger, almond milk, apple slices, and maple syrup to a mixing device.
2. Mix on high speed until everything combines into a creamy liquid.
3. Cool in the fridge for a few minutes before pouring into a glass.

Suggested Usage:

Sip this once each day, perhaps in the morning, to help ease general discomfort from swelling and support smoother tummy function.

Important Cautions:

Do not try this if you know you react badly to moringa or ginger, as it could cause upset. Always check with a health expert if you have ongoing issues.

Gentle Joint Soother Oil

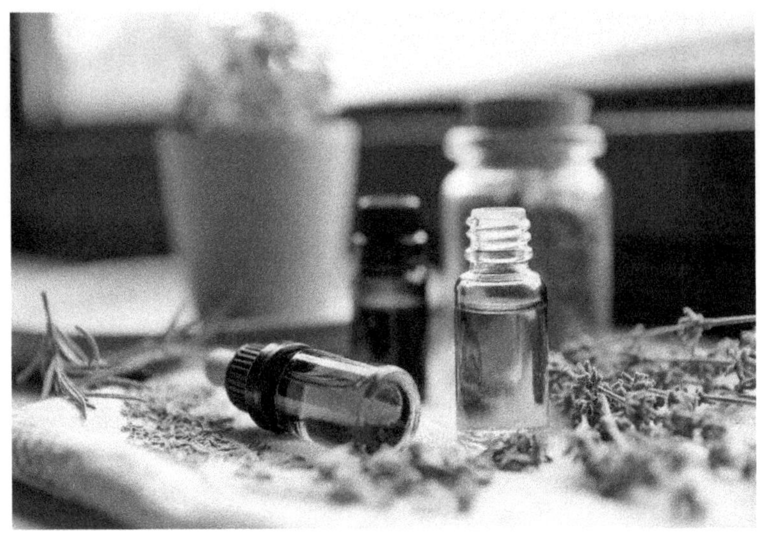

What You'll Need:

- 1 tablespoon pure black seed oil (nigella sativa)
- 5–6 drops frankincense essential oil (Boswellia variety works beautifully)

Steps to Prepare:

Simply pour the black seed oil into a small glass bowl or clean dropper bottle, add the frankincense drops, and swirl or shake gently until fully combined. That's it—no heat, no waiting.

Suggested Usage:

Warm a few drops between your palms, then massage gently into sore knees, hands, shoulders, or anywhere joints feel stiff. Apply morning and evening for steady relief. Let the oil soak in fully; a little goes a long way.

Important Cautions:

Keep away from broken or irritated skin. Always do a small patch test on the inside of your wrist first and wait 24 hours to rule out sensitivity. If you're pregnant, nursing, or on medication, check with your healthcare provider before use. Store in a cool, dark place and use within 6 months for best potency.

Warming Spice Blend Defense Drink

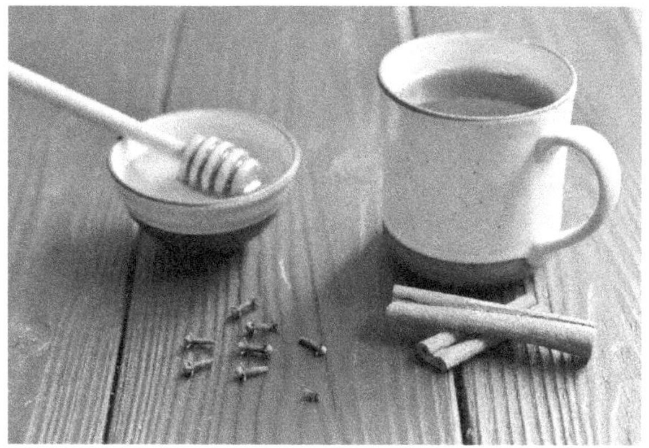

What You'll Need:

- A few whole cloves (about 4)
- One small piece of cinnamon bark
- A spoonful of natural sweetener like honey
- A mug of hot water

Steps to Prepare:

1. Heat the water until it's just starting to bubble, then add the cloves and cinnamon.
2. Let it gently simmer on low heat for around 8-10 minutes to draw out the flavors.
3. Pour through a fine mesh to remove the solids, mix in the sweetener while it's still warm, and allow it to reach a comfortable temperature.

Suggested Usage:

Enjoy one full mug each day to help support your body's natural ability to stay strong against everyday challenges.

Important Cautions:

Skip this if you know you're sensitive to spices like these, as it could cause discomfort. Always check with a health expert if you're unsure or have ongoing health concerns.

Calming Mist for Restful Nights

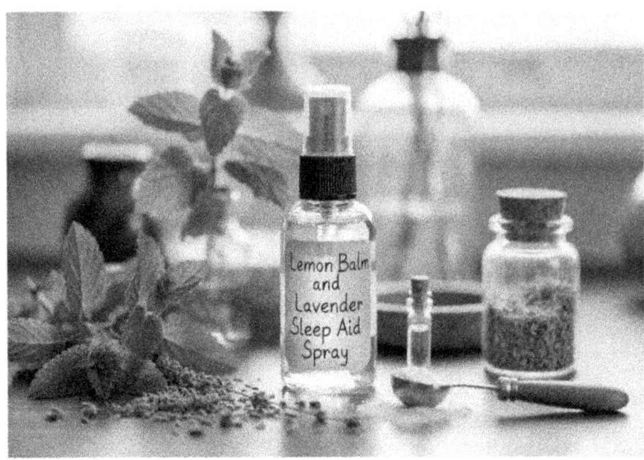

What You'll Need:

- 8 drops of lemon balm oil (from the plant known for its soothing effects)
- 12 drops of lavender oil (a gentle floral extract)
- 1 cup of pure, filtered water
- 1 tablespoon of natural alcohol-free dispersant (like a mild herbal extract solvent)

Steps to Prepare:

1. Pour the water into a clean glass spray container.
2. Add the lemon balm and lavender oils, followed by the dispersant to help everything blend smoothly.
3. Secure the lid and gently swirl the bottle to combine the mixture evenly.

Suggested Usage:

Lightly mist your bed linens or the air around your sleeping area about 30 minutes before bedtime to create a relaxing atmosphere.

Important Cautions:

Always do a small patch test on your inner arm to check for any irritation, and avoid direct contact with eyes or open wounds. Consult a healthcare provider if you're pregnant or have allergies.

Nourishing Blend for Feminine Balance Tea

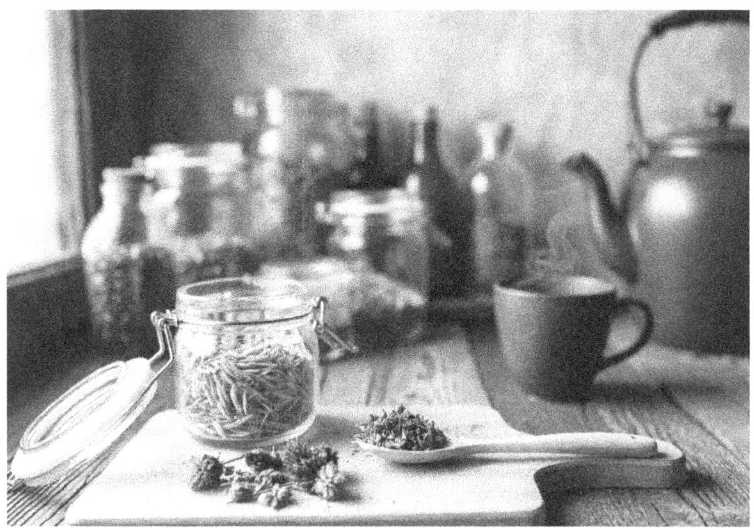

What You'll Need:

- 1 tablespoon dried oat straw
- 1 tablespoon dried red clover flowers
- 8 ounces boiling water

Steps to Prepare:

1. Add the oat straw and red clover flowers to a mug or teapot.
2. Pour the boiling water over the herbs and cover to keep the heat in.
3. Allow it to infuse for 15 minutes.
4. Filter out the plant material and sip while warm.

Suggested Usage:

Have one cup each day to help maintain even hormone levels and ease monthly cycle discomfort.

Important Cautions:

Skip this if you're expecting a baby or nursing. Consult a doctor if you have any health conditions.

Spicy Root Infusion for Achy Joint Soothing

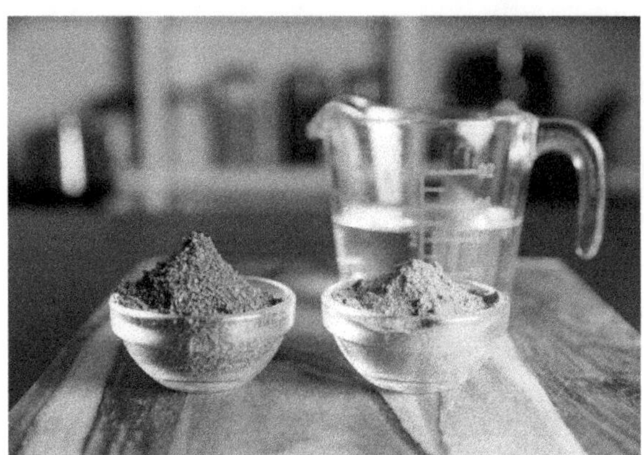

What You'll Need:

- 1 tablespoon ground red chili spice
- 1 tablespoon golden spice root powder
- 1/2 cup mild vegetable oil (like from olives)

Steps to Prepare:

1. Combine the red chili spice and golden spice root powder in a jar with the oil, stirring well to blend.
2. Place the jar in a sunny spot or near a gentle heat source for 48 to 72 hours, giving it a shake once or twice a day to help the flavors merge, then filter out the solids using a fine cloth or strainer.

Suggested Usage:

Gently rub a small amount onto areas with muscle tension or stiff joints for temporary comfort.

Important Cautions:

Avoid using on cuts, rashes, or sensitive areas to prevent discomfort; test a tiny patch on your skin first if you're unsure.

Calming Herb Duo Pills

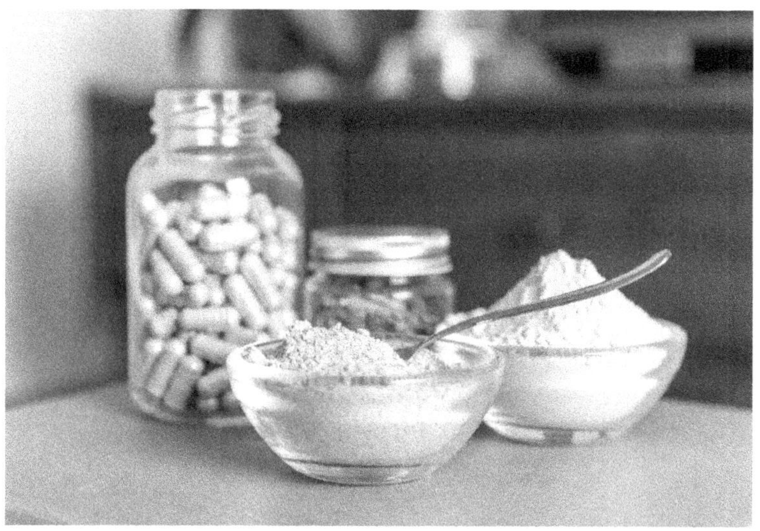

What You'll Need:

- 1 tablespoon of powdered centella (gotu kola) leaves
- 1 tablespoon of powdered winter cherry (ashwagandha) root
- Blank pill shells

Steps to Prepare:

1. Combine the centella powder and winter cherry powder in a small bowl, stirring until evenly blended.
2. Spoon the blend into the pill shells, packing them gently but firmly, then seal each one.

Suggested Usage:

Swallow one pill each day with water to help ease feelings of worry and tension.

Important Cautions:

Steer clear of this if you're expecting a baby or breastfeeding.

Peppermint and Elder Blossom Nasal Clearing Inhalation

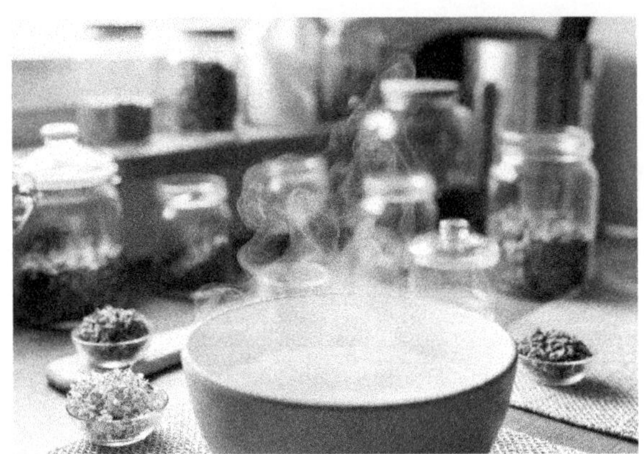

What You'll Need:

- 1 heaping teaspoon of dried elder blossoms
- 1 heaping teaspoon of dried mint leaves
- A large bowl filled with freshly boiled water

Steps to Prepare:

1. Pour the hot water into your bowl and let it cool just enough to avoid burns.
2. Sprinkle the dried blossoms and leaves into the water, stirring gently to mix.
3. Drape a clean towel over your head to create a tent over the bowl, then lean in and breathe deeply through your nose for about 5-10 minutes.

Suggested Usage:

Try this gentle vapor method up to two times each day to help open blocked nasal paths and soothe irritated tissues.

Important Cautions:

Skip this if you deal with any lung or breathing troubles, as the hot mist might make things worse. Always test the heat first to prevent skin discomfort.

Honeyed Citrus-Spice Cleanse Beverage

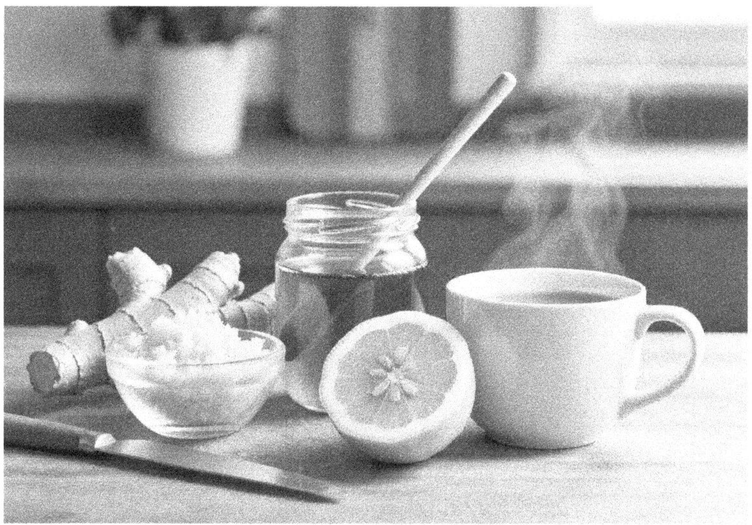

What You'll Need:

- 1 tablespoon minced fresh ginger root
- Juice squeezed from half a lemon (about 1 tablespoon)
- 1 tablespoon pure honey
- 1 cup of comfortably hot water

Steps to Prepare:

1. Add the minced ginger root, lemon juice, and honey to a mug.
2. Pour in the hot water and mix gently until the honey fully blends in.

Suggested Usage:

Enjoy this beverage right after waking up to energize your system and support natural body cleansing.

Important Cautions:

Skip this if you're sensitive to ginger or have related reactions.

Golden Spice Serenity Drink

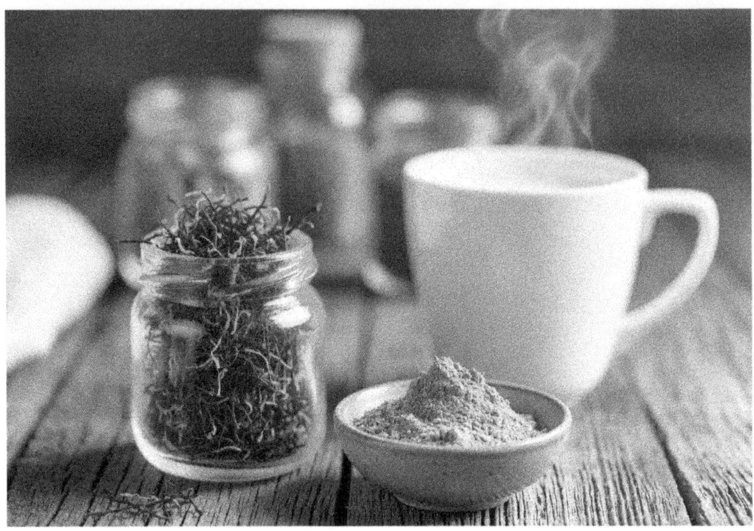

What You'll Need:

- A pinch of saffron strands (about 1/4 teaspoon)
- Ground cardamom (around 1/2 teaspoon)
- One cup of heated milk (dairy or plant-based like almond)

Steps to Prepare:

1. Let the saffron strands soak in the heated milk for roughly five minutes to release their color and flavor.
2. Mix in the ground cardamom, give it a good stir, and sip right away.

Suggested Usage:

Enjoy this beverage daily to help brighten your outlook and ease daily pressures.

Important Cautions:

Steer clear if you're expecting or have a known reaction to saffron.

Cleansing Herbal Infusion with Burdock and Dandelion

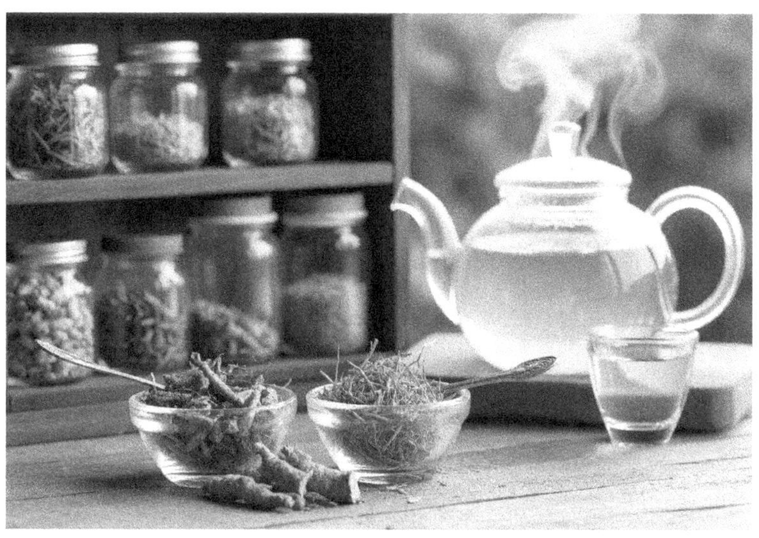

What You'll Need:

- 1 teaspoon dried burdock root
- 1 teaspoon dried dandelion root
- 2 cups boiling water

Steps to Prepare:

1. Add the burdock and dandelion roots to a heat-safe container.
2. Pour in the boiling water and cover to keep the heat in.
3. Allow the mixture to soak for 8-12 minutes.
4. Pour through a mesh strainer to remove the plant pieces, then sip warm.

Suggested Usage:

Enjoy one cup daily to help support liver cleansing and encourage clearer skin.

Important Cautions:

Skip this if you're pregnant, as it may not be suitable.

Calming Herbal Soak for Peaceful Rest

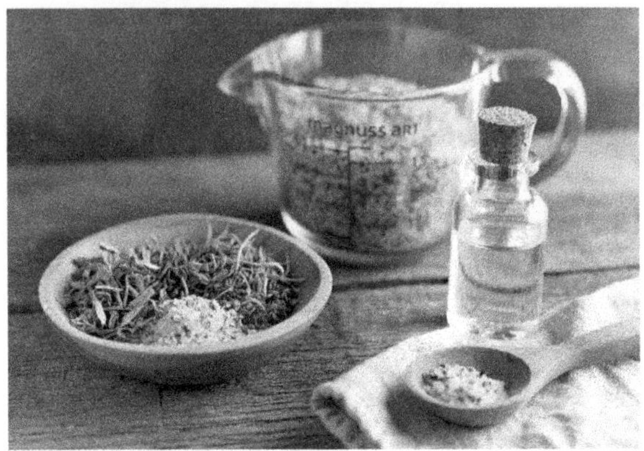

What You'll Need:

- 1 tablespoon of dried passionflower leaves
- 1 tablespoon of dried valerian rhizome
- 1 cup of magnesium-rich bath salts (like Epsom)
- 1 tablespoon of melted coconut carrier oil

Steps to Prepare:

1. In a small bowl, combine the dried herbs with the bath salts until evenly distributed.
2. Drizzle in the melted oil and stir gently to create a moist, aromatic blend that holds together lightly.

Suggested Usage:

Draw a comfortably warm tub of water, sprinkle in the mixture, and relax in it for about 20 to 30 minutes right before heading to bed. This helps unwind your mind and body for a more restful evening.

Important Cautions:

Skip this if you notice any skin irritation from valerian or if your blood pressure tends to run low, as it might enhance relaxing effects too much. Always test a small amount on your skin first.

Cooling Cucumber Aloe Mist for Skin Comfort

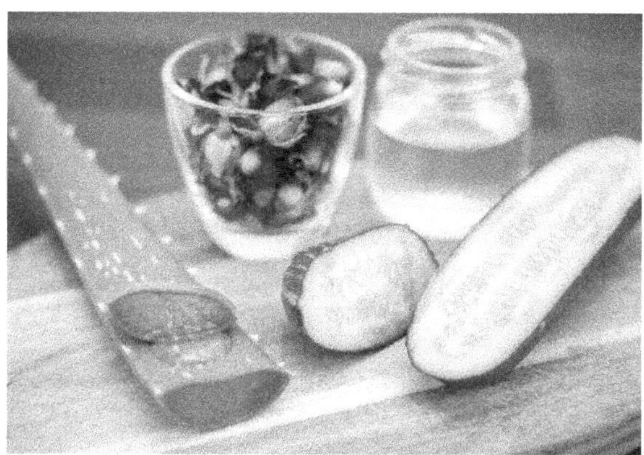

What You'll Need:

- One half of a fresh cucumber, ready to puree
- Two tablespoons of gel scooped from an aloe vera leaf
- Half a cup of gentle rose-infused water

Steps to Prepare:

1. Start by pureeing the cucumber in a food processor until it's a smooth liquid.
2. In a clean container, stir the pureed cucumber together with the aloe gel and rose water until fully combined.
3. Funnel the blend into a clean misting bottle and keep it chilled in your refrigerator for freshness.

Suggested Usage:

Lightly spritz onto areas where your skin feels hot from sun exposure or bothered by minor irritations to help cool and ease discomfort.

Important Cautions:

Before full use, apply a small amount to an inconspicuous spot on your arm and wait a day to ensure no sensitivity occurs.

Golden Spice Drink for Stomach Relief

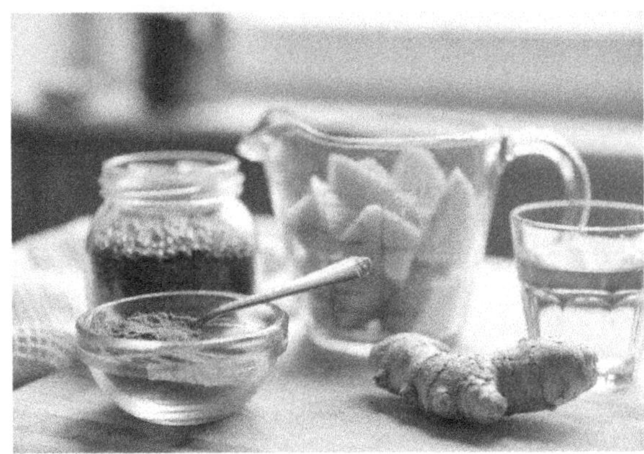

What You'll Need:

- 1/4 teaspoon ground turmeric
- A 1-inch piece of fresh ginger, peeled
- 1/2 cup mango pieces
- 1/2 cup plain water
- 1 teaspoon flax seeds

Steps to Prepare:

1. Roughly chop the ginger into smaller bits.
2. Place the turmeric, ginger, mango, water, and flax seeds into a blender.
3. Mix on high speed until everything combines into a creamy liquid.
4. Let it cool in the refrigerator for 10 minutes before serving.

Suggested Usage:

Sip this beverage roughly half an hour prior to eating to help calm stomach swelling and aid in smooth food processing.

Important Cautions:

Steer clear of this if you experience any adverse reactions to the spices or other items listed.

Adaptogen Blend Capsules for Daily Calm and Vitality

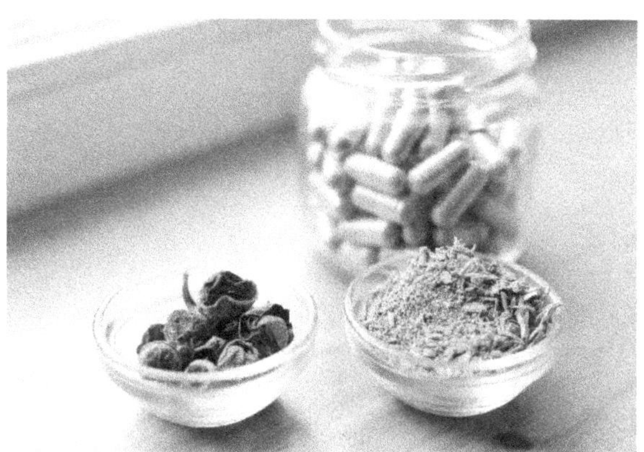

What You'll Need:

- 1 teaspoon of dried schisandra fruit
- 1 teaspoon of dried rhodiola rhizome
- Blank gelatin or vegetarian capsules

Steps to Prepare:

1. Crush the schisandra fruit and rhodiola rhizome into a fine dust using a mortar and pestle or a small grinder.
2. Scoop the blended dust into the capsules until they're full, then seal them securely.

Suggested Usage:

Swallow one capsule first thing each day to help ease tension and boost your stamina throughout the morning.

Important Cautions:

Steer clear of this if you're expecting a baby, and always check with your doctor before starting, especially if you're on any prescriptions.

Herbal Defense Blend Syrup

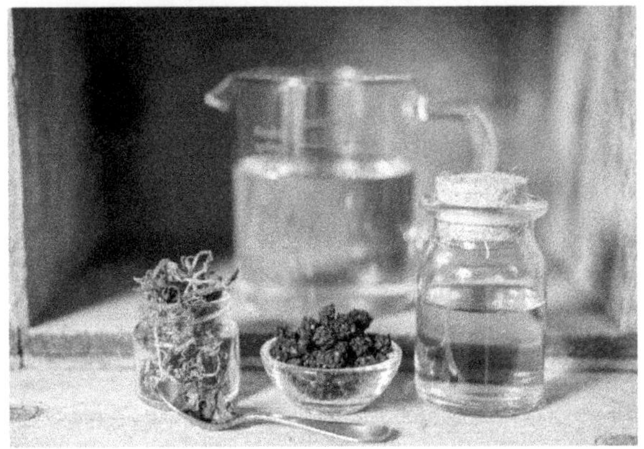

What You'll Need:

- 1 spoonful of dried purple coneflower root
- 1 spoonful of dried black elder fruits
- 1 cup of natural bee nectar
- 2 cups of fresh spring water

Steps to Prepare:

1. Gently heat the purple coneflower root and black elder fruits in the water over low flame for about half an hour.
2. Filter out the solids, then stir the warm liquid into the bee nectar until fully combined.
3. Pour into a clean glass container and let it cool before sealing.

Suggested Usage:

Consume a small spoonful each day to help strengthen your body's natural protections.

Important Cautions:

Skip this if you have sensitivities to plants in the daisy family.

Spice Soother for Dental Discomfort

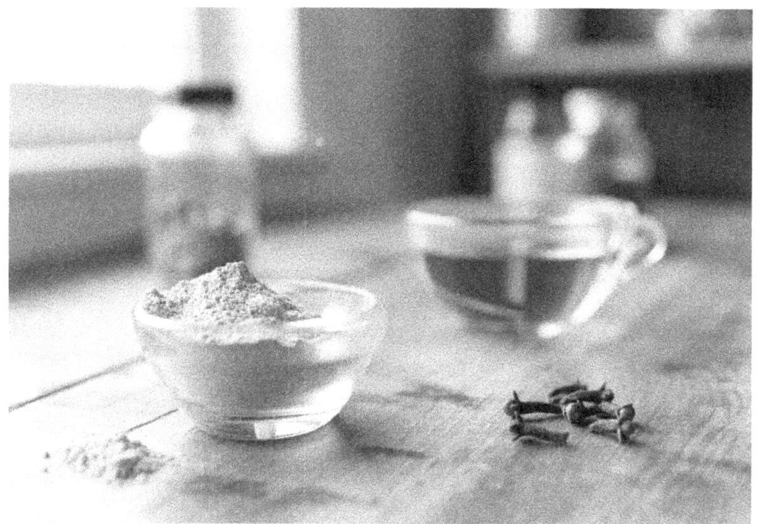

What You'll Need:

- A dash of powdered ginger (around 1/4 teaspoon)
- 3 dried cloves
- 1 tablespoon olive oil

Steps to Prepare:

1. Use a small grinder or mortar to turn the cloves into a fine powder.
2. Stir the ginger powder and clove powder together with the olive oil until it forms a smooth paste.

Suggested Usage:

Gently dab a bit of the paste onto the sore spot in your mouth using a clean cotton stick for short-term ease.

Important Cautions:

Don't swallow any of the paste. Test a tiny bit on your skin first to make sure you don't have a reaction to the spices.

Calming Root and Leaf Blend for Stress Ease

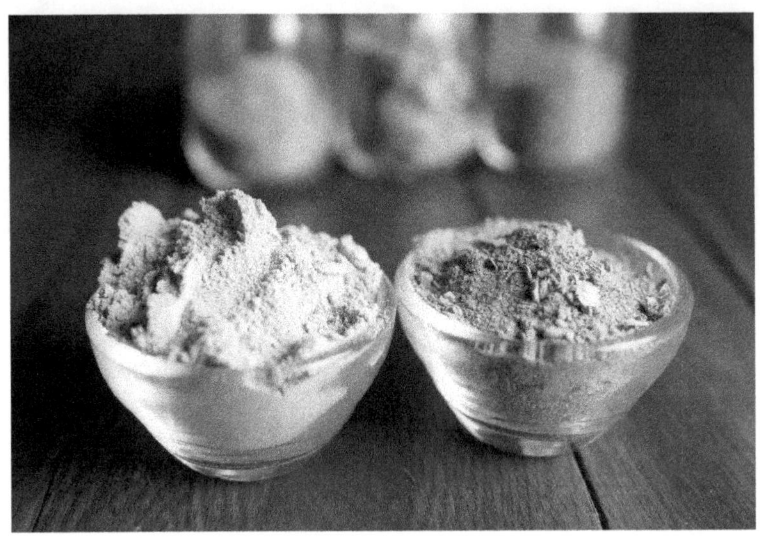

What You'll Need:

- One teaspoon of powdered ashwagandha root
- One teaspoon of ground holy basil leaves (also known as tulsi)

Steps to Prepare:

1. Pour the powders into a clean dish.
2. Blend them together until fully combined.

Suggested Usage:

Stir half a teaspoon into a cup of heated water or your favorite warm beverage each day to help soothe nerves and promote relaxation.

Important Cautions:

Speak with a healthcare professional prior to starting if you're expecting or using treatments for hormone-related conditions.

Soothing Blend Syrup for Scratchy Throats

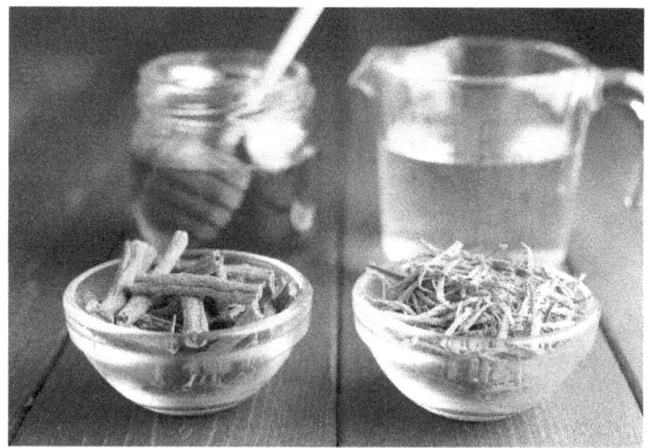

What You'll Need:

- 1 tablespoon of dried licorice root pieces
- 1 tablespoon of dried marshmallow root shreds
- 1 cup of pure honey
- 2 cups of fresh water

Steps to Prepare:

1. Place the licorice and marshmallow roots in a pot with the water, and heat it until it starts simmering gently for about 25 minutes.
2. Remove from heat, filter out the plant bits using a fine mesh, and stir the remaining liquid into the honey until fully blended.

Suggested Usage:

Spoon out 1 teaspoon as needed throughout the day to ease throat discomfort.

Important Cautions:

Skip this if you have issues with elevated blood pressure or if you're expecting a baby. Always check with a doctor before trying new herbal mixes.

Spicy Nectar Vitality Tonic

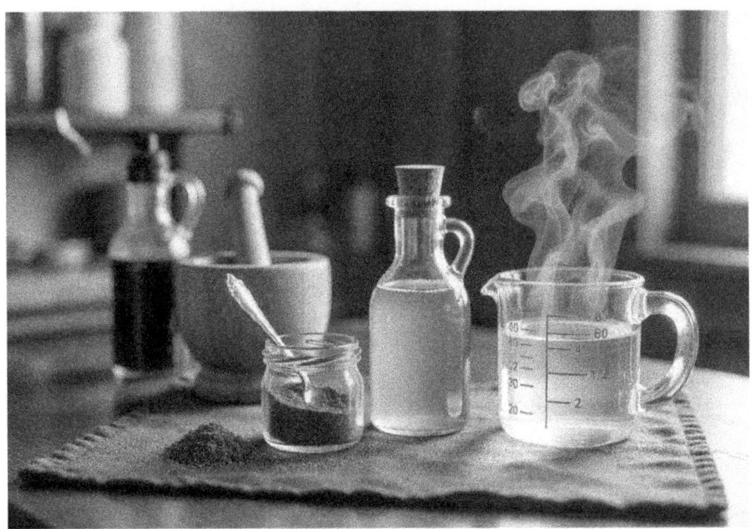

What You'll Need:

- 1/2 teaspoon ground red pepper
- 2 tablespoons raw honey
- 8 ounces hot water

Steps to Prepare:

1. Start by blending the ground red pepper into the hot water until it's fully mixed in.
2. Stir in the raw honey until everything combines smoothly.

Suggested Usage:

Sip this mixture prior to exercise or movement to help support healthy circulation.

Important Cautions:

Skip this if you react poorly to heat in foods or deal with stomach discomfort.

Calming Blossom and Herb Soothing Brew

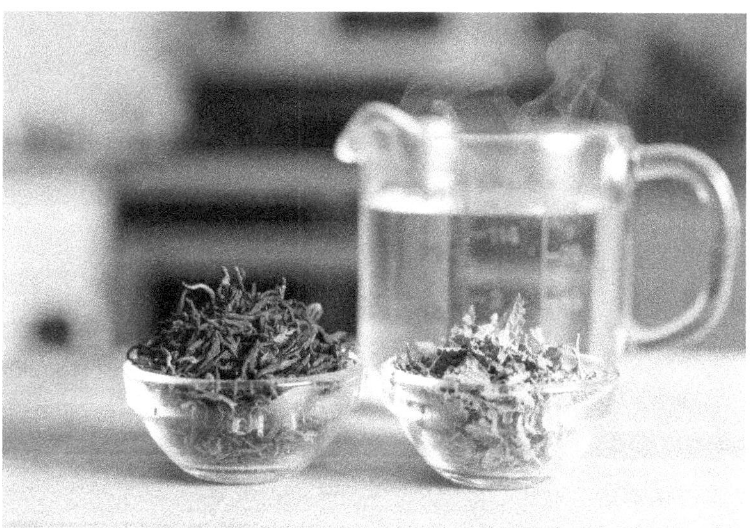

What You'll Need:

- 1 teaspoon of dried hibiscus flowers
- 1 teaspoon of dried lemon balm foliage
- 2 cups of freshly boiled water

Steps to Prepare:

1. Place the flowers and foliage in a teapot or mug.
2. Pour the boiled water over them and let it sit covered for about 8 minutes.
3. Filter out the plant material before enjoying.

Suggested Usage:

Sip on this brew up to twice a day to help ease tension and promote relaxation.

Important Cautions:

This may lead to slight sleepiness in some people. Skip it before driving or using heavy equipment.

Soothing Spice Blend Drink

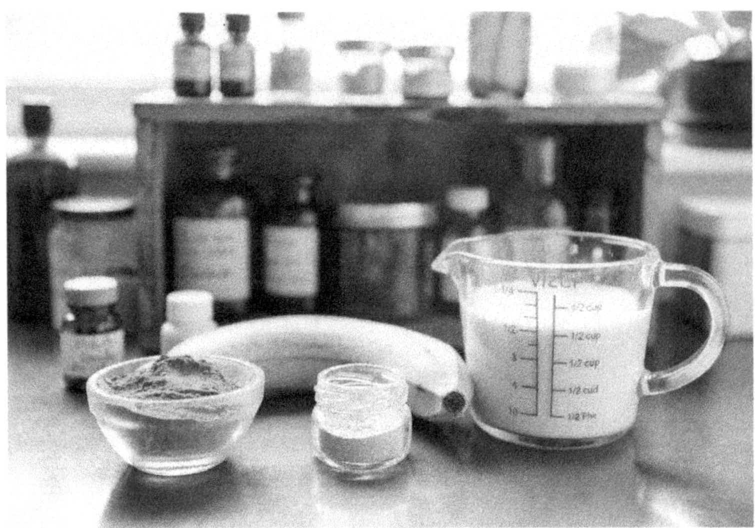

What You'll Need:

- 1/2 teaspoon powdered cinnamon
- 1/4 teaspoon powdered ginger
- 1 ripe banana
- 1/2 cup oat milk

Steps to Prepare:

1. Add everything to a blender and mix until creamy and well combined.

Suggested Usage:

Enjoy one serving each day to help ease body swelling and support comfort.

Important Cautions:

Limit intake if you are expecting a baby or nursing, as higher amounts may not be suitable.

Garlic and Oregano Infusion for Lung Comfort

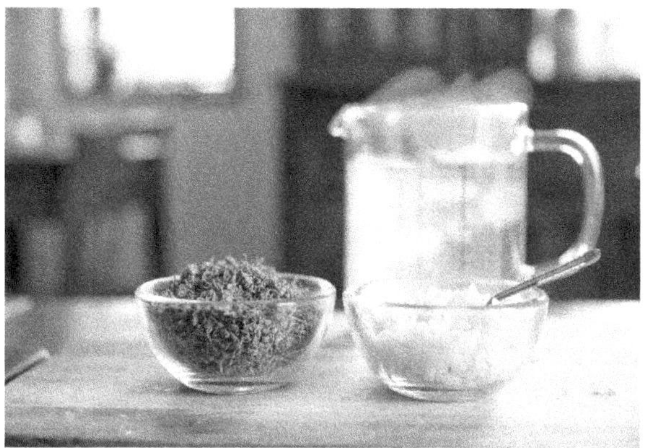

What You'll Need:

- 2 teaspoons of dried oregano leaves
- 2 small garlic cloves, finely minced
- 8 ounces of boiling water

Steps to Prepare:

1. Place the minced garlic and oregano in a heat-safe mug.
2. Carefully pour the boiling water over the mixture.
3. Cover and allow it to sit for about 12 minutes to draw out the natural essences.
4. Filter out the solids using a fine mesh strainer, then sip while still warm.

Suggested Usage:

Enjoy this warm brew once or twice a day to help ease breathing and support clear airways during times of stuffiness.

Important Cautions:

Skip this if you have sensitivities to garlic or oregano. Check with a healthcare provider before use if you're expecting a baby, nursing, or taking blood-thinning medications, as garlic might affect clotting.

Lavender and Eucalyptus Headache Relief Oil

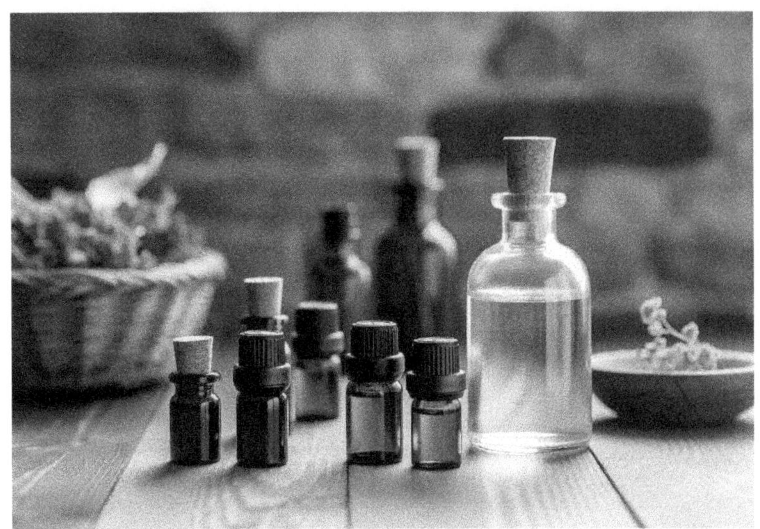

What You'll Need:

- 5 drops of lavender essential oil
- 5 drops of eucalyptus essential oil
- 1 tablespoon of a base oil, such as jojoba or almond oil

Steps to Prepare:

1. Pour the base oil into a small glass container.
2. Add the lavender and eucalyptus essential oils.
3. Stir or shake lightly until everything combines evenly.

Suggested Usage:

Dab a few drops onto your fingertips and rub softly onto the sides of your forehead when discomfort arises.

Important Cautions:

Steer clear of getting this near your eyes or any tender areas to prevent irritation.

Berry Boost Defense Mix

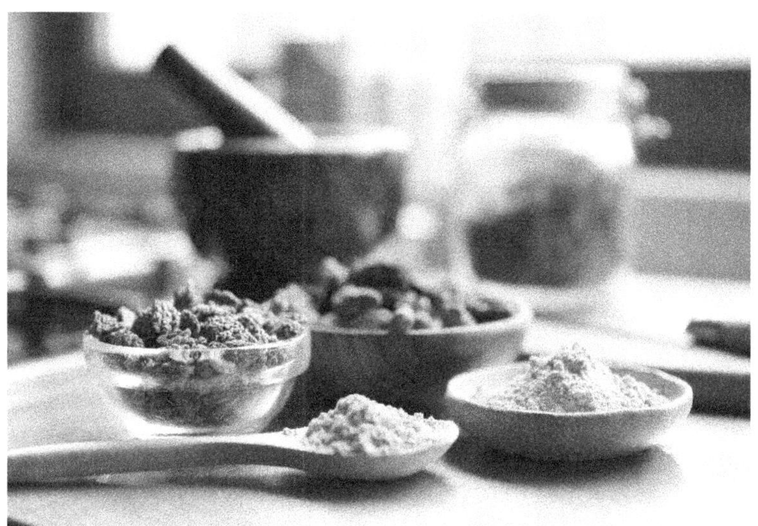

What You'll Need:

- 2 tablespoons dried wolfberries (also known as goji berries)
- 1/2 tablespoon ground sweet root (licorice)
- 1 tablespoon finely milled echinacea root

Steps to Prepare:

1. Place all the items in a clean blender or spice grinder.
2. Blend until you get a smooth, even dust-like texture.
3. Store the mix in a sealed jar away from light and heat.

Suggested Usage:

Stir a small spoonful into your morning drink, like juice or a fruit blend, to help keep your body's natural defenses strong, especially during busy or low-energy days.

Important Cautions:

Skip this if you're expecting a baby or dealing with elevated blood pressure. Always check with a doctor if you have ongoing health concerns.

Soothing Herbal Infusion for Easing Worry

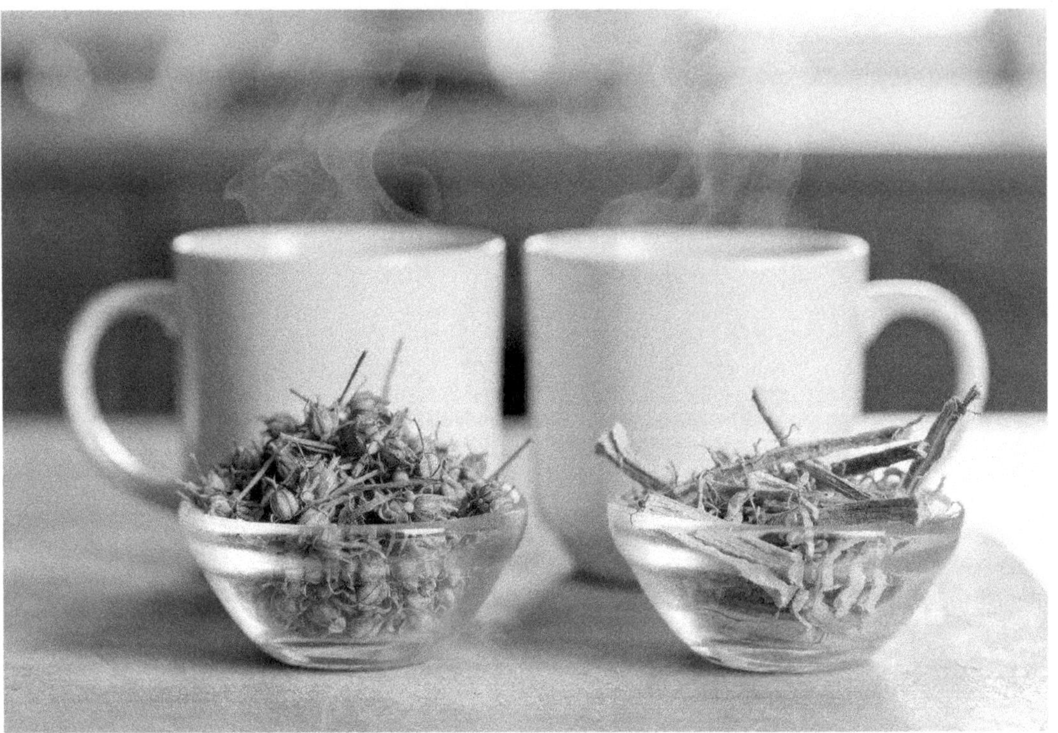

What You'll Need:

- 1 teaspoon of dried hypericum flowers (commonly known as St. John's wort)
- 1 teaspoon of dried valerian rhizome
- 2 mugs of freshly boiled water

Steps to Prepare:

1. Place the hypericum flowers and valerian rhizome into a teapot or heat-safe container.
2. Pour the boiled water over the herbs and cover to keep the warmth in.
3. Allow the mixture to infuse for about 10 to 20 minutes, depending on how strong you prefer it.
4. Filter out the plant material using a fine mesh strainer or cloth.

Suggested Usage:

Sip this infusion in the evening, ideally an hour before bedtime, to help promote a sense of relaxation and support restful nights.

Important Cautions:

Consult a healthcare provider before use, especially if you're on medications for mood or mental health, as hypericum can interact with them. Not recommended during pregnancy or while breastfeeding without professional advice. Stop use if you notice any skin sensitivity to sunlight or other unusual reactions.

Propolis and Elder Blossom Wellness Blend

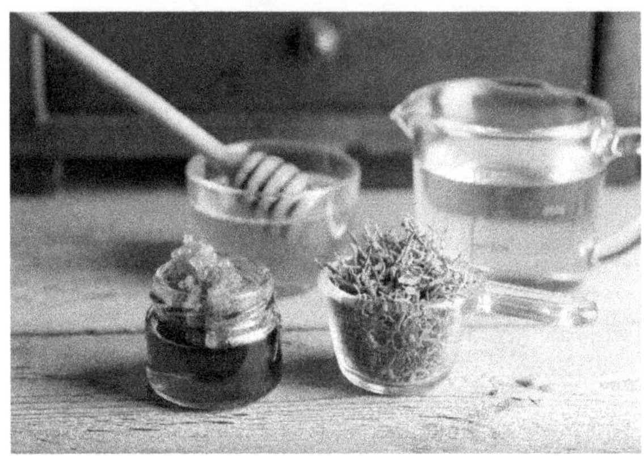

What You'll Need:

- 1 tablespoon of propolis tincture from bees
- 1 tablespoon of dried elder blossoms
- 1/2 cup of raw honey
- 1 cup of boiling water

Steps to Prepare:

1. Pour the boiling water over the dried elder blossoms in a heat-safe container and let it sit covered for around 10 minutes to draw out the natural essences.
2. Strain out the blossoms, then stir in the propolis tincture and honey until everything blends smoothly into a thick mixture.
3. Let it cool, then store in a clean jar in a cool spot.

Suggested Usage:

Spoon out 1 teaspoon each day to help support your body's natural defenses, especially during seasonal changes.

Important Cautions:

Skip this if you're sensitive to bee-related items, as it could cause reactions. Always check with a health expert if you have concerns.

Nourishing Herbal Rinse for Thicker Locks

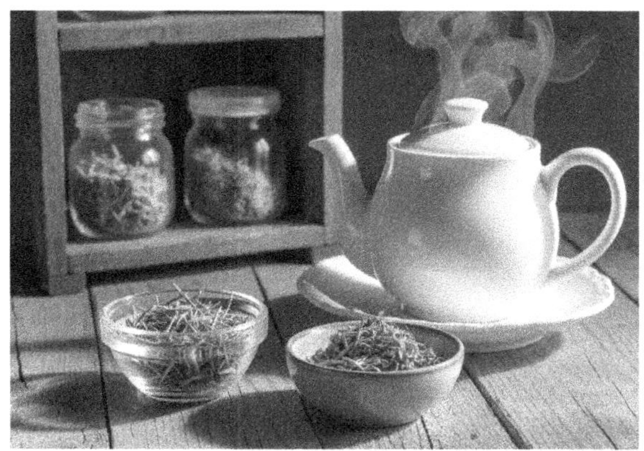

What You'll Need:

- 1 tablespoon of dried rosemary leaves
- 1 tablespoon of dried lemon balm leaves
- 2 cups of freshly boiled water

Steps to Prepare:

1. Place the rosemary and lemon balm leaves in a heat-safe container.
2. Pour the boiled water over the leaves and cover the container to keep the heat in for about 15 minutes.
3. Filter out the leaves using a fine mesh strainer or cloth, then allow the liquid to cool to a comfortable temperature.

Suggested Usage:

Pour the rinse over your clean, wet hair after your regular wash, massaging it gently into the scalp. No need to rinse it out afterward. Try this routine two to three times each week to support stronger, fuller hair over time.

Important Cautions:

Always do a small skin test on your inner arm first—apply a bit of the rinse and wait 24 hours to see if any irritation occurs. Avoid if you have known allergies to these plants, and consult a doctor if you're pregnant or have scalp conditions.

Mullein and Licorice Root Cough Syrup

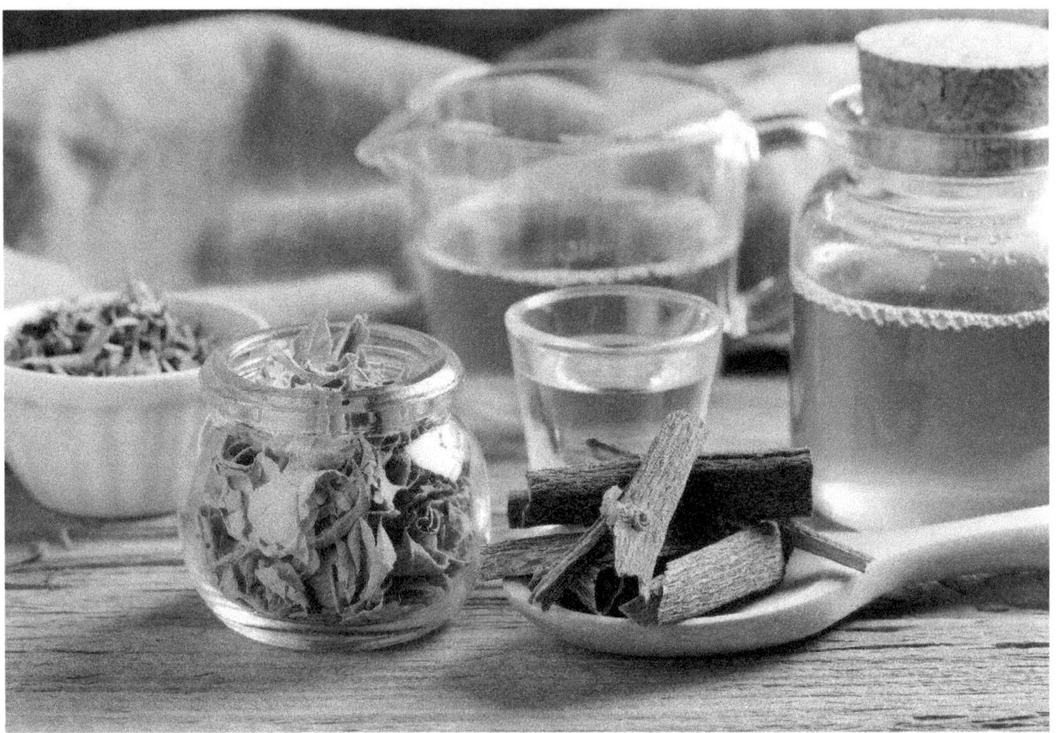

What You'll Need:

- 1 tablespoon dried mullein leaves
- 1 tablespoon dried licorice root
- 1 cup honey (raw or local works best for extra soothing benefits)
- 1 cup water

Steps to Prepare:

1. Place the dried mullein leaves and licorice root in a small pot with the water.
2. Bring the mixture to a gentle boil, then lower the heat and let it simmer for 15 minutes. This draws out the helpful compounds from the herbs.
3. Turn off the heat and strain the liquid through a fine mesh strainer or cheesecloth into a clean bowl or jar, pressing gently on the herbs to extract as much liquid as possible. Discard the herbs.
4. While the strained liquid is still warm (but not hot), stir in the honey until it fully dissolves.
5. Allow the syrup to cool completely, then transfer it to a clean glass jar or bottle with a tight lid. Store in the refrigerator for up to 2 weeks.

Suggested Usage:

Take 1 teaspoon of the syrup every 2 to 3 hours as needed to help ease coughs and soothe your throat. Shake the jar gently before each use. Adults can enjoy it straight or mixed into warm water or tea.

Important Cautions:

Avoid this remedy during pregnancy or if you have high blood pressure, kidney issues, or an allergy to licorice. Licorice root can affect fluid balance in the body when used in larger amounts or for long periods.

Spice Infusion for Tummy Comfort

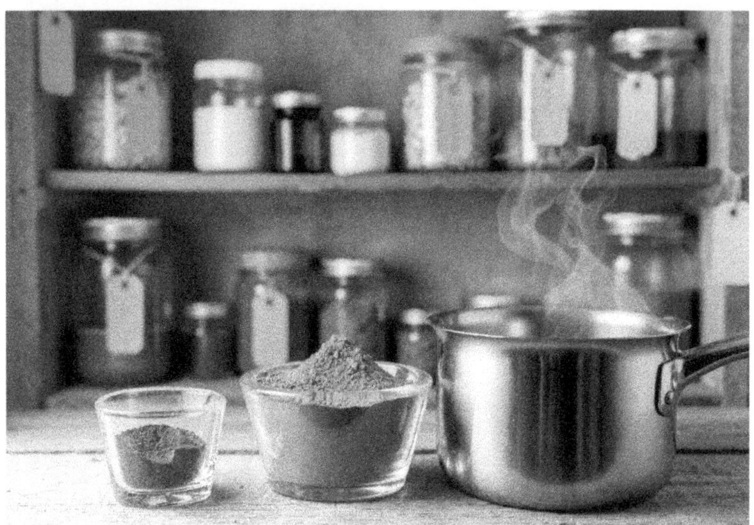

What You'll Need:

- 1/4 teaspoon powdered clove
- 3/4 teaspoon powdered cinnamon bark
- 8 ounces heated water (not boiling)

Steps to Prepare:

1. Pour the heated water into a mug.
2. Add the powdered spices directly into the water.
3. Mix vigorously for about 30 seconds to blend everything evenly.

Suggested Usage:

Sip this gently about 20 minutes prior to eating to help soothe your stomach and support smooth food processing.

Important Cautions:

Use sparingly if you're expecting a baby or have a delicate digestive system, as too much could cause discomfort.

Refreshing Spice and Citrus Cleanse Drink

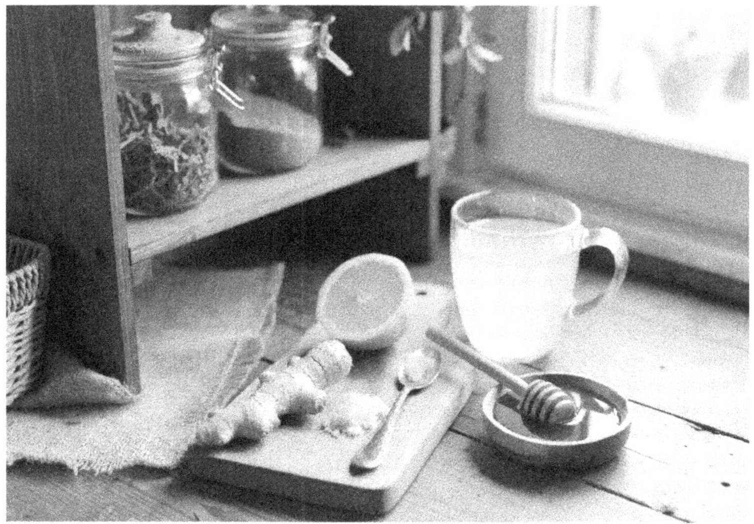

What You'll Need:

- A small piece of fresh ginger root (about 2 cm), finely chopped
- 1 tablespoon of juice from a fresh lemon
- 1 teaspoon of natural honey
- 1 cup of hot water (not boiling)

Steps to Prepare:

1. Place the chopped ginger in a mug and pour the hot water over it. Let it sit for about 10 minutes to infuse.
2. Pour the mixture through a fine mesh strainer into another cup, then stir in the lemon juice and honey until well mixed.

Suggested Usage:

Sip this beverage each morning to help support your body's natural cleansing process.

Important Cautions:

Skip this if you have sensitivities to lemon or ginger.

Minty Breath Revitalizer Mist

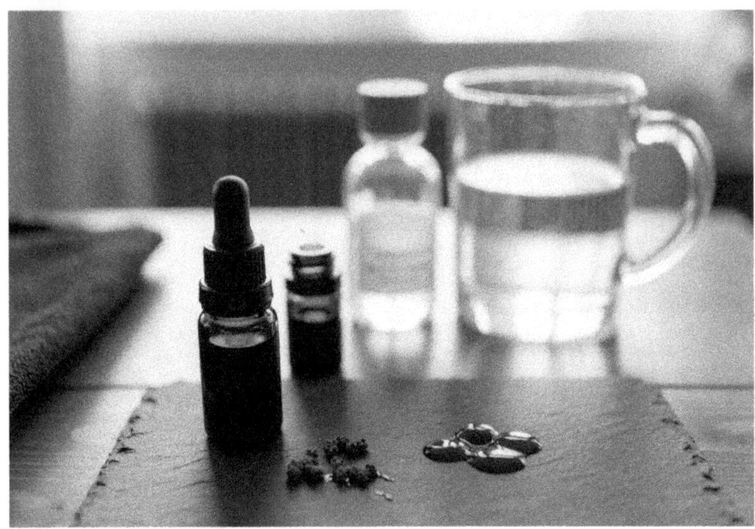

What You'll Need:

- 4 drops of peppermint oil (from essential oils)
- 6 drops of spearmint oil (from essential oils)
- 1 tablespoon of witch hazel without alcohol
- 2 tablespoons of clean, filtered water

Steps to Prepare:

1. Pour all the items into a tiny bottle with a spray top.
2. Give it a good mix by swirling gently.

Suggested Usage:

Mist a couple of sprays inside your mouth whenever you want a quick refresh.

Important Cautions:

Don't drink it. Make sure it doesn't get near your eyes.

Golden Spice Facial Glow Treatment

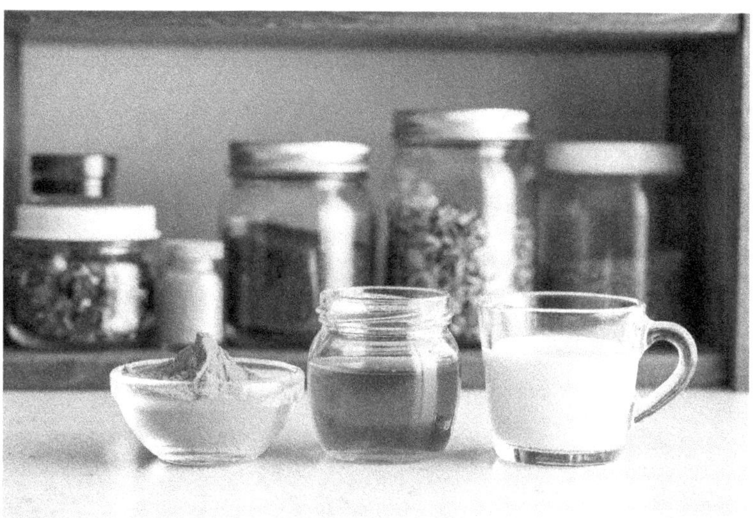

What You'll Need:

- 1 teaspoon ground turmeric
- 1 teaspoon raw honey
- 1 teaspoon plain milk

Steps to Prepare:

1. Combine the items in a small dish until they form a creamy mixture.
2. Spread the blend gently across your face, avoiding the eyes.
3. Let it sit for about 10 minutes to absorb.
4. Wash off using lukewarm water and pat dry.

Suggested Usage:

Apply this once every seven days to help enhance your skin's natural radiance.

Important Cautions:

Always do a small patch test on your arm before full use to check for any irritation.

Natural Blend for Clearer Skin

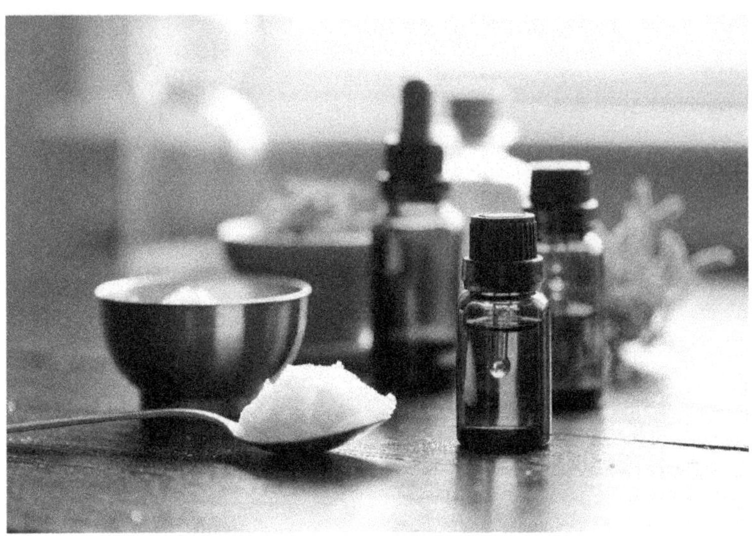

What You'll Need:

- One spoonful of virgin coconut oil
- A couple of drops of pure tea tree essential oil

Steps to Prepare:

1. Combine the coconut oil with the tea tree drops in a small container.
2. Stir gently until well blended for even distribution.
3. Dab the mixture onto spots where breakouts often appear.

Suggested Usage:

Apply this blend to your skin once each day to help manage pimples and promote a smoother complexion.

Important Cautions:

Keep away from your eyes to prevent stinging. Test on a small patch of skin first, as it might bother those with delicate skin types.

Relaxing Evening Beverage for Better Rest

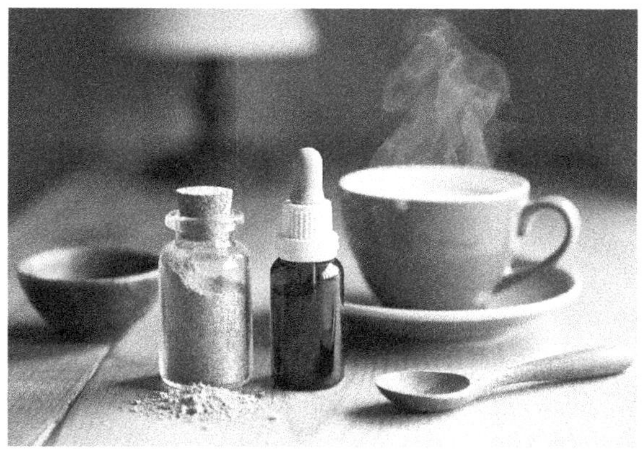

What You'll Need:

- 1 teaspoon ground ashwagandha root
- 1 drop pure lavender oil
- 1 cup heated milk or a plant-based option like almond or oat milk

Steps to Prepare:

1. Warm up your choice of milk in a small pot or microwave until it's comfortably hot but not boiling.
2. Sprinkle in the ashwagandha root and add the lavender oil.
3. Whisk or blend everything together for about a minute to combine evenly.
4. Pour into your favorite cup and sip slowly as part of your wind-down routine.

Suggested Usage:

Enjoy this drink about an hour before turning in for the night to encourage a calm mind and deeper slumber.

Important Cautions:

Skip this if you're pregnant, breastfeeding, or using any drugs that make you sleepy, as it might increase drowsiness. Always check with a doctor if you have health conditions or take other medicines.

Herbal Infusion for Nourishing Hair and Promoting Thickness

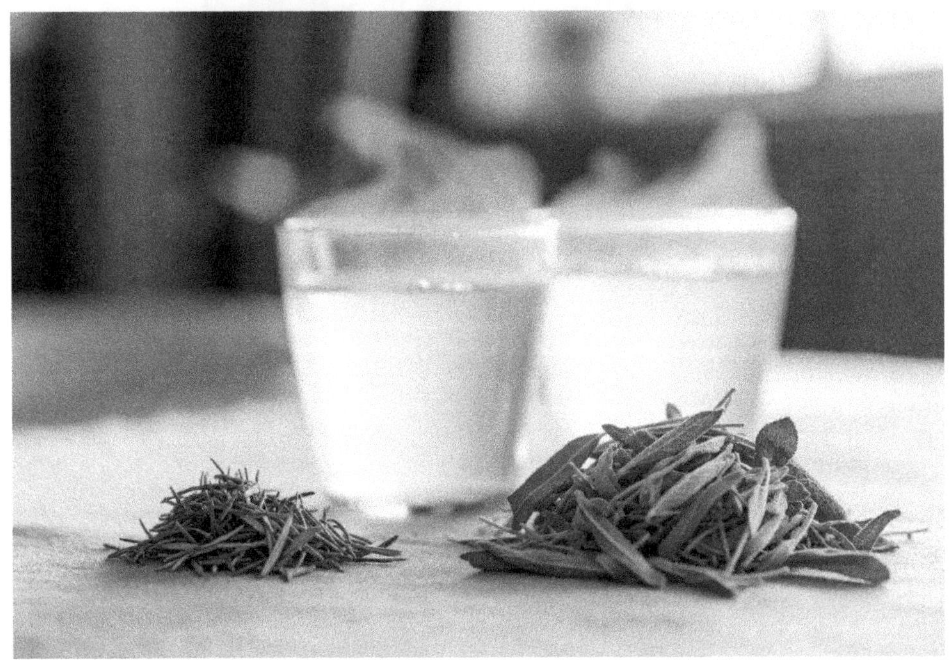

What You'll Need:

- A small handful of dried rosemary leaves (about one large spoonful)
- An equal amount of dried sage leaves
- Two full cups of freshly boiled water

Steps to Prepare:

1. Place the rosemary and sage in a heat-safe container and pour the hot water over them.
2. Cover the mixture and let it sit undisturbed for around 20 minutes to draw out the natural essences.
3. Filter out the plant material using a fine mesh or cloth, then allow the liquid to cool to a comfortable temperature.

Suggested Usage:

After washing your hair as usual, pour the cooled infusion over your scalp and strands, massaging gently. Let it air dry without rinsing out. Aim for application every few days, such as two or three times weekly, to support healthier, fuller-looking hair over time.

Important Cautions:

Always do a small skin patch test on your arm first to check for any sensitivity or reaction. Avoid if you have known plant allergies, and consult a healthcare provider if you're pregnant or have scalp conditions.

Berry Boost Soothing Mixture for Chills

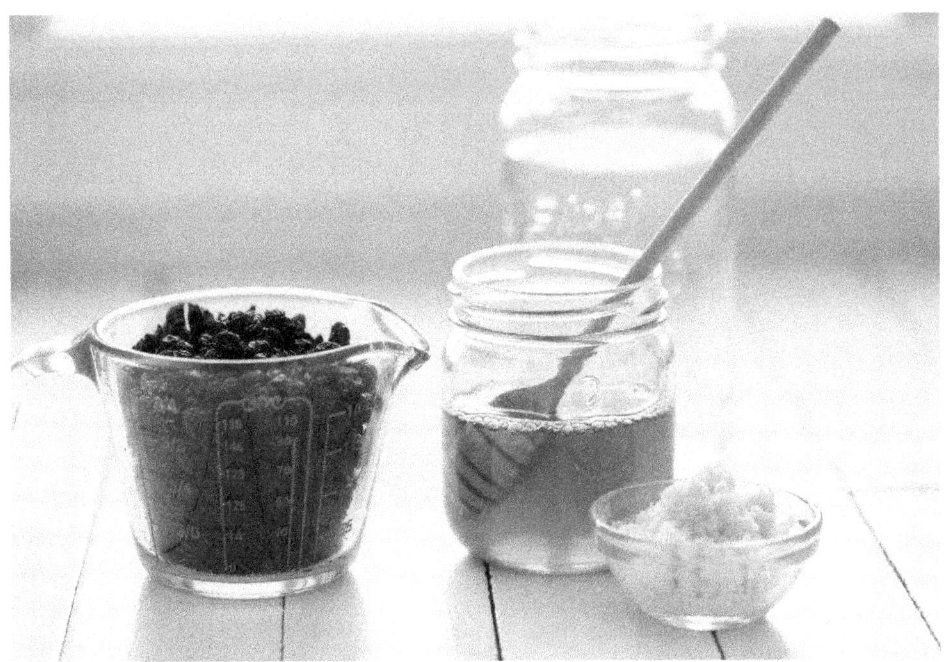

What You'll Need:

- 3/4 cup dried elderberries
- 1/3 cup raw honey
- 2 teaspoons fresh grated ginger root
- 2 cups filtered water

Steps to Prepare:

1. In a small pot, combine the elderberries, ginger, and water, then bring to a gentle boil over medium heat.
2. Reduce the heat and let it bubble softly for about 30 minutes, stirring now and then to release the flavors.
3. Remove from the stove, allow it to cool down to room temperature, then press through a fine mesh sieve to separate the liquid from the solids.
4. Stir in the honey until it fully dissolves, and pour the mixture into a clean glass jar for storage in the fridge.

Suggested Usage:

Spoon out 1 teaspoon every few hours when feeling under the weather, up to four times a day, to help ease discomfort.

Important Cautions:

Avoid giving this to kids younger than 1 year old due to honey content; consult a doctor for anyone with health conditions or if symptoms persist.

Calming Herbal Blend for Easing Worry

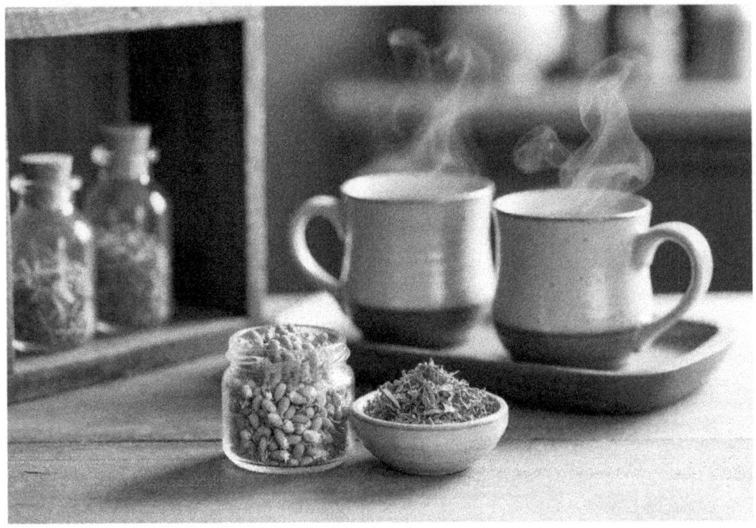

What You'll Need:

- 1 heaping teaspoon of dried chamomile blooms
- 1 heaping teaspoon of dried lemon balm greens
- 2 mugs of freshly boiled water

Steps to Prepare:

1. Combine the chamomile and lemon balm in a heat-safe container.
2. Add the hot water and cover to keep the warmth in.
3. Allow the mixture to rest undisturbed for 10 to 15 minutes to draw out the flavors.
4. Pour through a fine mesh to remove the plant bits, then sip while warm.

Suggested Usage:

Have a serving when tension builds up during the day or right before sleep to help unwind and settle the mind.

Important Cautions:

Skip this if you react badly to plants like ragweed or others in the daisy group. Always check with a doctor if you're unsure about allergies or if you're pregnant.

Evergreen Soak for Body Cleansing

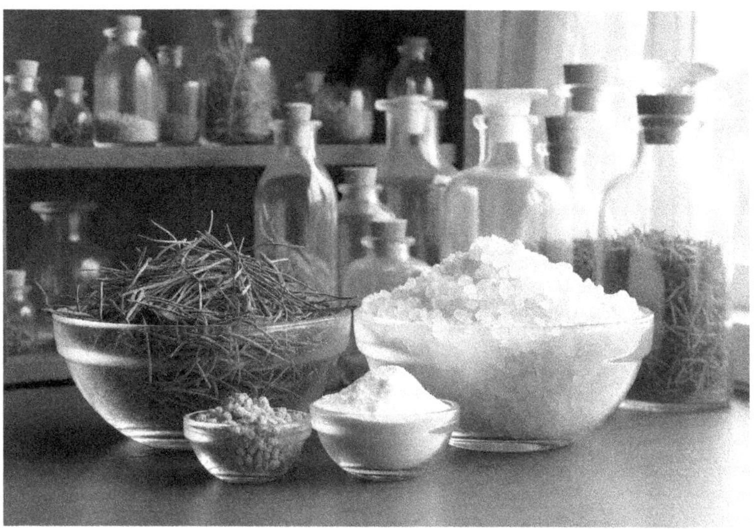

What You'll Need:

- 1 handful of fresh or dried pine twigs (about 3/4 cup)
- 1/3 cup of lightly bruised juniper fruits
- 1 1/2 cups of magnesium sulfate crystals
- 1/3 cup of sodium bicarbonate

Steps to Prepare:

1. Heat the pine twigs and juniper fruits in a pot of simmering water for around 15 minutes to draw out their natural essences.
2. Filter out the solids, then pour the warm liquid into your tub water, stirring in the crystals and bicarbonate until they dissolve.

Suggested Usage:

Relax in the tub for 15-25 minutes to help your body release built-up impurities and feel refreshed.

Important Cautions:

Skip this if you're expecting a baby or if your skin tends to react easily to new things.

Cooling Veggie and Plant Blend Calming Lotion

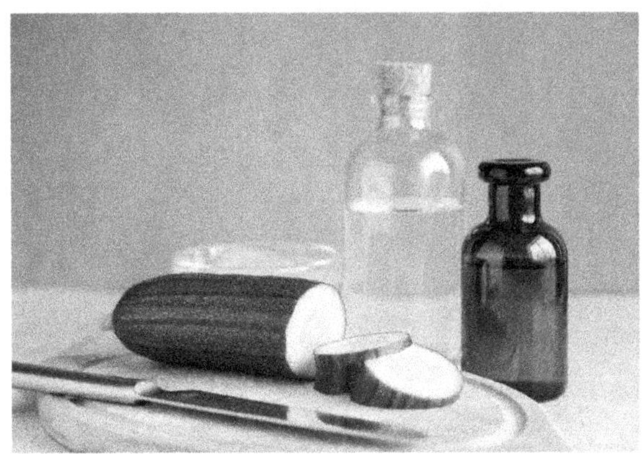

What You'll Need:

- One medium-sized fresh cucumber, pureed
- Two tablespoons of fresh aloe vera extract
- Half a teaspoon of olive oil

Steps to Prepare:

1. Puree the cucumber in a food processor until smooth, then filter out the liquid using a fine mesh strainer or cheesecloth.
2. Combine the cucumber liquid with the aloe vera extract in a small bowl.
3. Stir in the olive oil until everything blends into a smooth mixture.
4. Store in a clean jar in the fridge for up to three days.

Suggested Usage:

Apply a thin layer to affected areas like sun-exposed or itchy skin, and leave it on for about 20 minutes before rinsing with cool water. Great for easing discomfort after too much time outdoors.

Important Cautions:

Skip this if you have sensitivity to olives or any plant-based oils. Always test a small patch on your arm first to check for reactions. Not for use on open wounds or if you're pregnant without consulting a doctor.

Tropical Blend for Gut Comfort

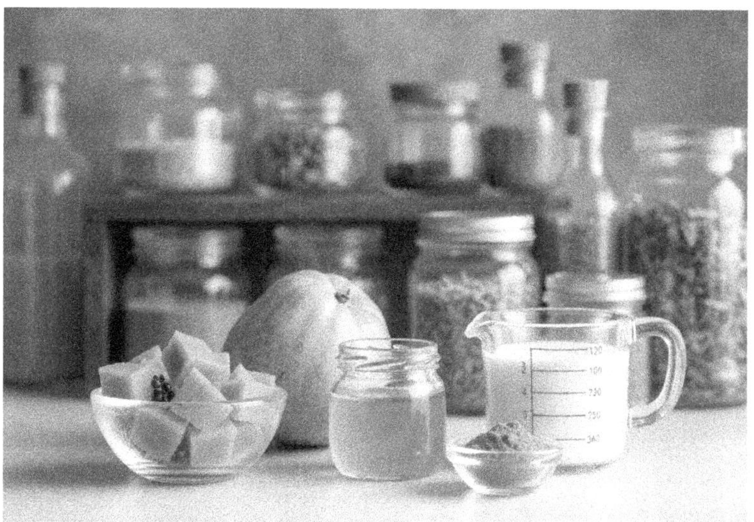

What You'll Need:

- 1/2 cup cubed ripe papaya
- 1 tablespoon natural honey
- 1/2 cup light coconut milk
- 1/4 teaspoon ground turmeric

Steps to Prepare:

1. Add the papaya cubes, honey, turmeric, and coconut milk to a mixer.
2. Puree everything until it's creamy and uniform.
3. Pour into a glass and let it cool in the refrigerator for a bit.

Suggested Usage:

Sip this refreshing drink first thing after waking to help ease your stomach and promote smooth processing of food.

Important Cautions:

Skip this if you have sensitivities to tropical fruits or spices in the mix.

Revitalizing Blossom Facial Spritz

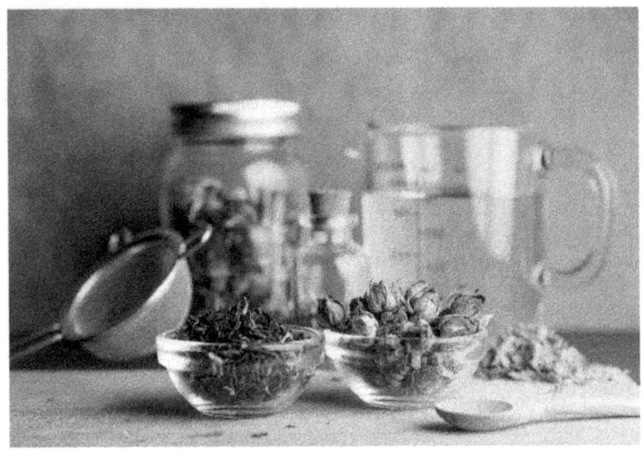

What You'll Need:

- 2 teaspoons of crushed hibiscus petals
- 1 teaspoon of dried rose buds
- 8 ounces of filtered water

Steps to Prepare:

1. Warm the water to a gentle simmer in a small pot.
2. Mix in the hibiscus petals and rose buds, then remove from heat and cover to let the mixture infuse for about 15 minutes.
3. Pour through a mesh strainer to remove the solids, allowing the liquid to cool completely.
4. Transfer the cooled infusion into a clean misting container for easy application.

Suggested Usage:

Lightly spray over your skin any time you want a quick burst of moisture and a soothing pick-me-up.

Important Cautions:

Apply a small amount to a discreet spot on your skin first to make sure there's no irritation or allergic response.

Honey Garlic Defense Elixir

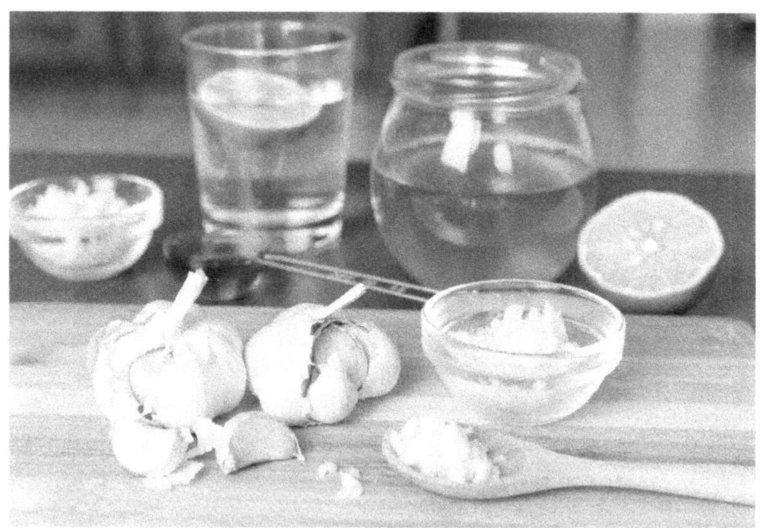

What You'll Need:

- 3 fresh garlic cloves, finely chopped
- 1/3 cup raw honey
- 2 teaspoons fresh lime juice

Steps to Prepare:

1. Mix the chopped garlic with the honey and lime juice in a small bowl.
2. Transfer the mixture to a clean glass container with a tight lid and allow it to rest at room temperature for a full day to blend flavors.

Suggested Usage:

Consume a small spoonful each morning to help strengthen your body's natural defenses.

Important Cautions:

Do not give to kids younger than 2 years, as honey can pose health risks for them.

Soothing Herbal Vapor for Nasal Congestion

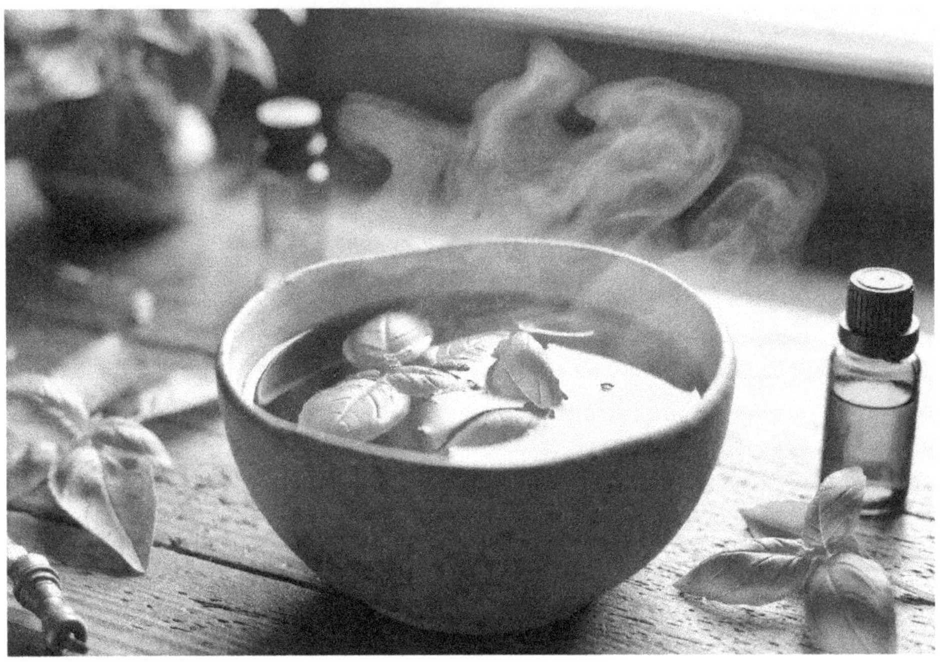

What You'll Need:

- A handful of fresh basil leaves (about 4-6)
- 4 drops of eucalyptus essential oil
- A large bowl filled with hot, freshly boiled water

Steps to Prepare:

1. Place the basil leaves into the bowl and drizzle the eucalyptus oil over them.
2. Carefully pour the hot water into the bowl, allowing the mixture to release its aromas.
3. Wait a moment for the steam to build, then position your face over the bowl (keeping a safe distance to avoid burns) and drape a towel over your head to trap the vapors.

Suggested Usage:

Breathe in the warm, scented steam slowly and deeply for around 8-12 minutes to help ease blocked nasal passages when dealing with sniffles or stuffiness from a common cold. Repeat up to twice a day as needed for comfort.

Important Cautions:

Keep away from young children under the age of 2, as the strong scents and heat could be overwhelming. Always test for skin sensitivity by diluting the oil first if there's any contact, and stop if you feel any discomfort like dizziness or irritation. Consult a doctor if symptoms persist or worsen.

Nut and Grain Skin Renewer

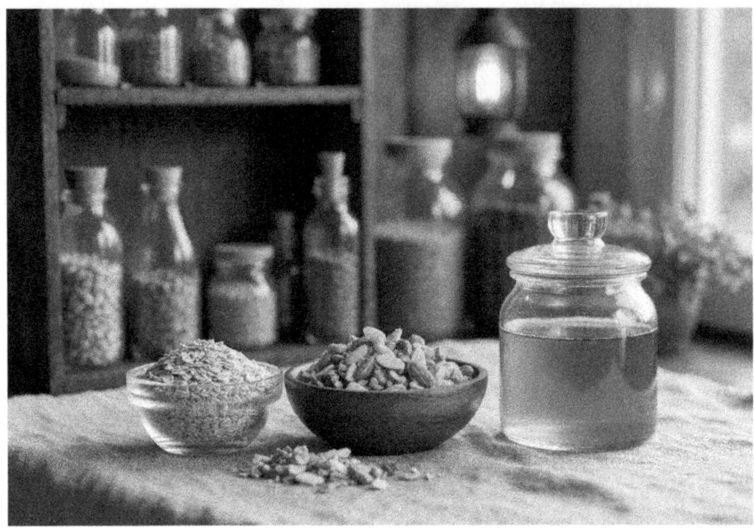

What You'll Need:

- 1 tablespoon finely milled oats
- 1 tablespoon crushed nut bits (like almonds)
- 1 tablespoon pure, raw honey

Steps to Prepare:

1. In a clean bowl, blend the milled oats with the crushed nuts until evenly mixed.
2. Add the honey and stir well to create a smooth, spreadable blend.

Suggested Usage:

Dampen your skin first, then apply the mixture and massage lightly in small circles over your face or body for a minute or two. Rinse with warm water. Try this routine a couple of times each week to help refresh and smooth your skin.

Important Cautions:

Before applying to larger areas, dab a small amount on your inner arm and wait a day to check for any skin reactions, particularly if you're sensitive to nuts.

Calming Herb Blend for Stress Reduction

What You'll Need:

- 2 teaspoons dried lemon balm leaves
- 1 teaspoon dried lavender buds
- 16 ounces freshly boiled water

Steps to Prepare:

1. Place the lemon balm leaves and lavender buds into a heat-safe mug or infuser.
2. Pour the boiled water over the herbs and cover to keep the aromas in.
3. Allow the mixture to infuse for 8 to 12 minutes, depending on how strong you like it.
4. Remove the herbs by straining, then sip slowly while warm.

Suggested Usage:

Enjoy a cup when tension builds up during the day or as part of your evening wind-down routine to promote relaxation.

Important Cautions:

Skip this if you're expecting a baby, as it might not be suitable. Always check with a doctor if you have health concerns.

Cayenne and Ginger Muscle Soother

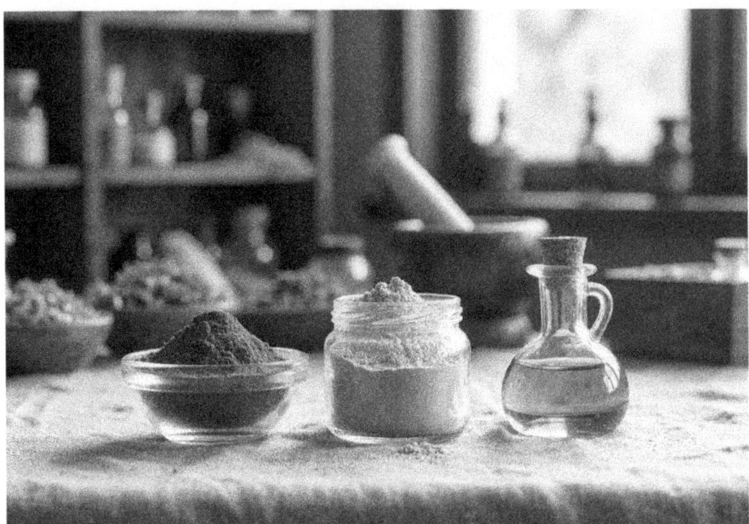

What You'll Need:

- 1 tablespoon cayenne pepper powder
- 1 teaspoon ginger powder
- 2 tablespoons olive oil

Steps to Prepare:

1. In a small bowl, stir the cayenne pepper powder and ginger powder into the olive oil until everything is well blended and smooth.
2. That's it—your rub is ready to use right away.

Suggested Usage:

Rub a small amount onto sore, tired muscles and massage in gentle circles. It offers quick, temporary comfort for everyday aches from activity or strain.

Important Cautions:

Never apply to cuts, scrapes, or broken skin. Wash your hands thoroughly after use, and keep it away from your eyes, nose, and mouth. If irritation occurs, rinse with cool water and discontinue use.

Citrus Revitalizing Foot Buff

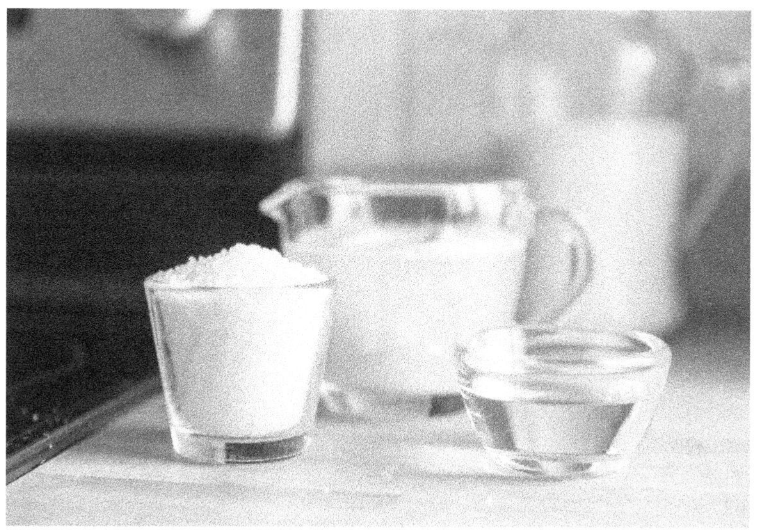

What You'll Need:

- Half a cup of coarse salt crystals
- Juice squeezed from one fresh lemon (roughly one tablespoon)
- One tablespoon of light vegetable oil

Steps to Prepare:

1. In a small bowl, blend the salt crystals with the fresh lemon juice and vegetable oil until you get a thick, spreadable mixture.
2. Gently massage the blend onto your feet in circular motions for about five minutes, then wash away with warm water.

Suggested Usage:

Apply this once a week to slough away rough patches and invigorate tired soles.

Important Cautions:

Skip this if there are any breaks in the skin on your feet to prevent irritation.

Stinging Nettle and Fresh Ginger Scalp Toner

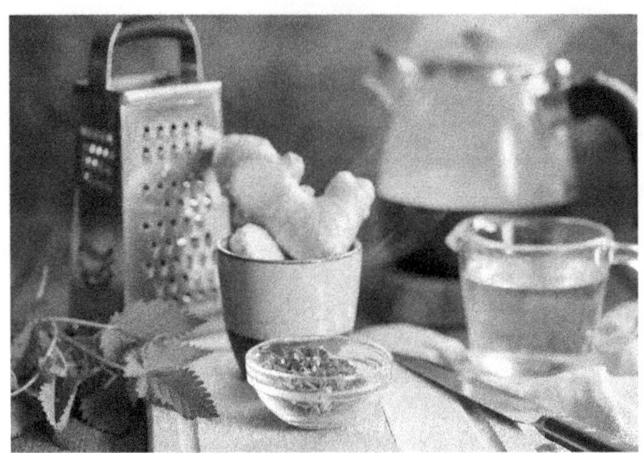

What You'll Need:

- 2 tablespoons chopped fresh stinging nettle leaves (or 1 tablespoon dried if fresh unavailable)
- 1-inch piece of fresh ginger root, grated
- 2 cups hot water (just off the boil)

Steps to Prepare:

1. Combine the nettle leaves and grated ginger in a heat-safe container.
2. Pour the hot water over the mixture and cover it to let the flavors infuse for about 20 minutes.
3. Filter the liquid through a fine mesh strainer or cloth to remove all plant bits.
4. Let it cool to room temperature before applying to your hair.

Suggested Usage:

Apply this toner to clean, damp hair once or twice weekly to help nourish the scalp and encourage vibrant, resilient strands.

Important Cautions:

Skip this if you know you're sensitive to stinging nettle or ginger, as it might cause skin irritation. Test a small amount on your arm first if unsure.

Refreshing Herb and Floral Face Spritz

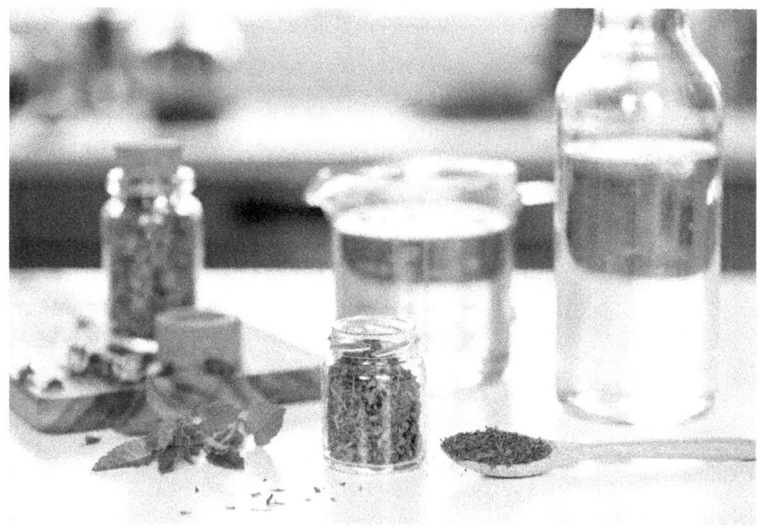

What You'll Need:

- 1 tablespoon dried peppermint foliage
- 1/4 cup rose-infused liquid
- 1/2 cup clean, filtered water

Steps to Prepare:

1. Soak the peppermint foliage in hot water for around 10 minutes to draw out its essence.
2. Filter the mixture to remove the solids, then blend in the rose-infused liquid and clean water.
3. Transfer the blend to a small bottle with a spray top for easy keeping.

Suggested Usage:

Lightly mist over your skin for a quick refresh when the weather feels warm.

Important Cautions:

Do not use it if you have reactions to peppermint or rose products.

Spicy Shield Brew

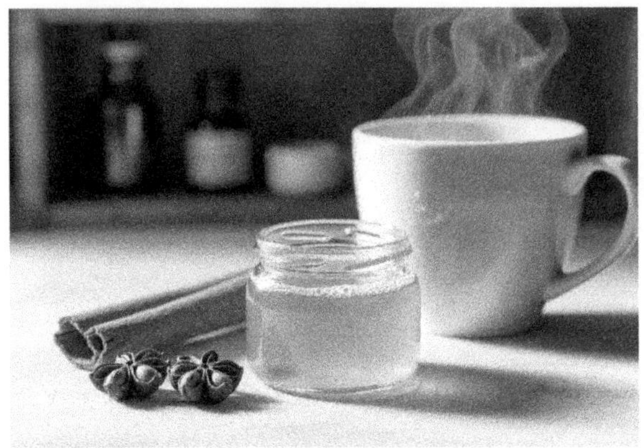

What You'll Need:

- 3 whole cloves
- A small piece of cinnamon bark (about 1 inch)
- 1 tablespoon of raw honey
- 1.5 cups of freshly boiled water

Steps to Prepare:

1. Place the cloves and cinnamon bark into a heat-safe mug or pot.
2. Pour the boiled water over them and let the mixture sit covered for about 8 minutes to draw out the flavors.
3. Remove the spices by pouring through a fine mesh strainer into your cup.
4. Stir in the honey until it dissolves completely, adjusting the amount if you prefer it sweeter.

Suggested Usage:

Sip on this brew every morning when sniffles are going around to help support your body's natural defenses.

Important Cautions:

Avoid this if you're taking medications that affect blood clotting, as it might interact with them. Always check with a doctor if you have health concerns.

Citrus Grass and Tea Cleansing Soak

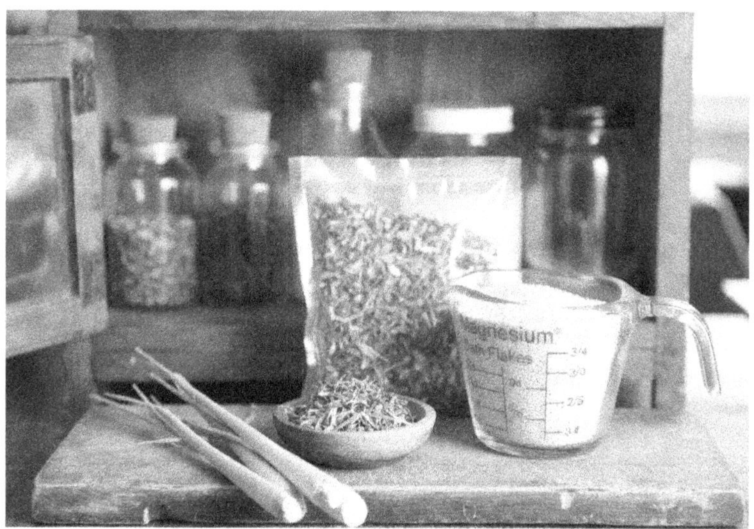

What You'll Need:

- 2 tablespoons chopped dried citrus grass (lemongrass)
- 1 bag of loose-leaf green tea
- 3/4 cup magnesium bath flakes (Epsom salt)

Steps to Prepare:

1. Tie the citrus grass and green tea bag together in a thin cloth pouch or piece of fabric.
2. Run warm water into your tub and sprinkle in the magnesium flakes, stirring gently until they dissolve.
3. Hang or place the pouch under the faucet as the tub fills, allowing the warm water to draw out the essences.

Suggested Usage:

Ease into the warm water and relax for about 15-25 minutes to help refresh and purify your body.

Important Cautions:

Steer clear if you have any known reactions to citrus grass or green tea components.

Soothing Green Veggie Face Blend

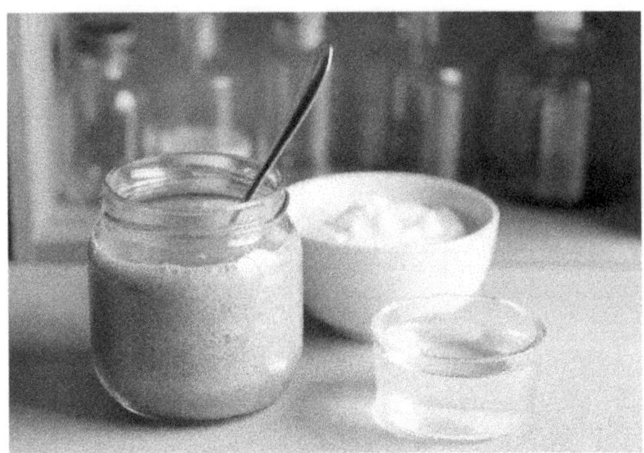

What You'll Need:

- One quarter of a fresh cucumber, blended smooth
- Three tablespoons of plain creamy yogurt
- Half a teaspoon of aloe vera gel

Steps to Prepare:

1. Puree the cucumber in a blender until it's a fine paste.
2. Combine the puree with the yogurt and aloe vera gel in a small bowl, stirring until evenly mixed.
3. Spread the blend gently over your clean face, avoiding the eyes.
4. Let it sit for about 10 to 20 minutes while you relax.
5. Gently wash away with lukewarm water and pat dry.

Suggested Usage:

Apply this blend to calm skin that's feeling hot or uncomfortable after time in the sun or from minor irritations. It's best used once or twice a week for a refreshing feel.

Important Cautions:

Test a small patch on your arm first to check for any skin reactions. Avoid if you have known sensitivities to milk-based items or fresh produce like cucumber. Consult a doctor if irritation persists.

Golden Spice Blend for Sore Spots

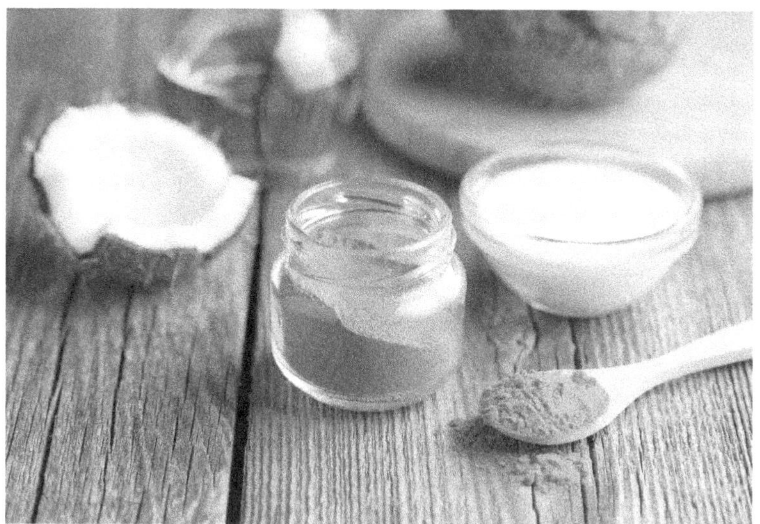

What You'll Need:

- 1 tablespoon ground turmeric
- 2 tablespoons pure coconut oil

Steps to Prepare:

1. Gently warm the coconut oil in a small dish until it softens, if needed.
2. Stir in the ground turmeric gradually to create a uniform mixture.
3. Allow the blend to set slightly for easier handling.

Suggested Usage:

Gently rub onto areas with discomfort, such as stiff knees or tense shoulders, and let it rest for about half an hour before rinsing with mild soap.

Important Cautions:

This blend can leave temporary yellow marks on fabric or your body. Do not use it on any broken or irritated skin.

Soothing Herbal Blend for Peaceful Slumber

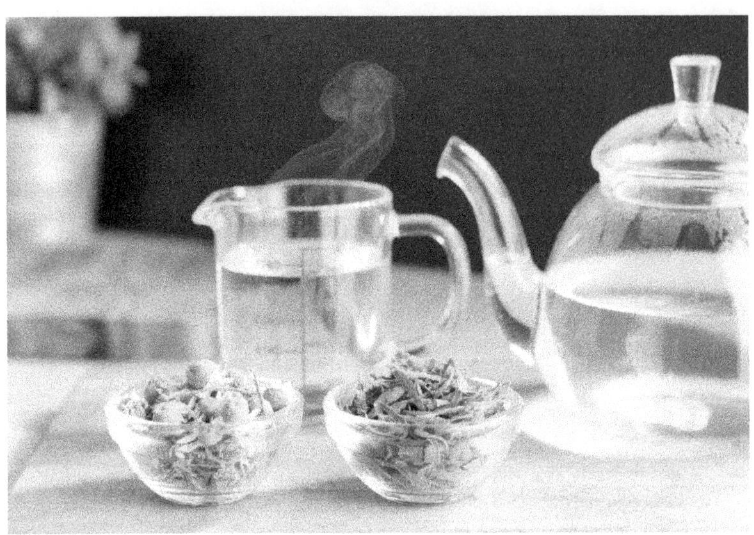

What You'll Need:

- 2 teaspoons of dried chamomile flowers
- 2 teaspoons of dried lemon balm leaves
- 8 ounces of freshly boiled water

Steps to Prepare:

1. Add the chamomile flowers and lemon balm leaves to a mug or teapot.
2. Pour the boiled water over the mixture and cover it to keep the warmth in.
3. Allow it to infuse for 8 to 12 minutes, then filter out the plant material.

Suggested Usage:

Enjoy a warm cup in the evening routine to encourage calm and support natural rest.

Important Cautions:

Skip this if you're expecting or feeding a baby, as it might not be suitable.

Tropical Fruit and Spice Soother for Better Digestion

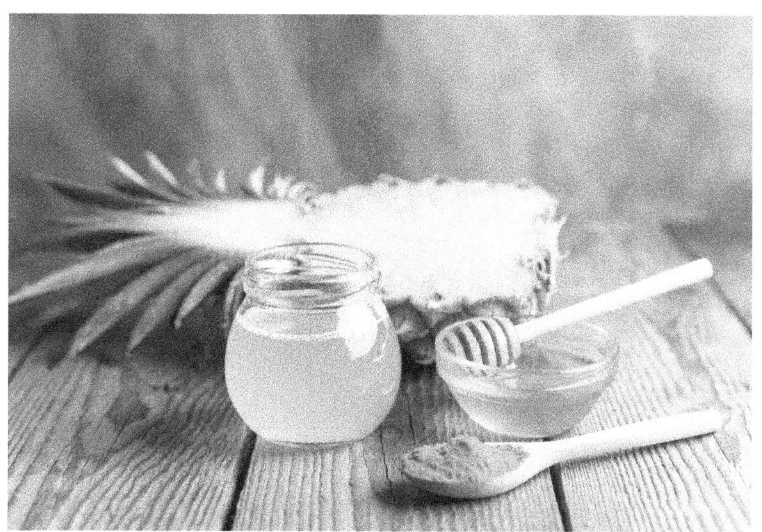

What You'll Need:

- 4 ounces of juice squeezed from ripe pineapple
- A quarter teaspoon of ground turmeric
- 2 teaspoons of raw honey

Steps to Prepare:

1. Pour the pineapple juice into a small bowl or cup.
2. Sprinkle in the turmeric and drizzle the honey on top.
3. Whisk vigorously for about a minute until the mixture is smooth and the spices fully blend in.

Suggested Usage:

Enjoy a small glass following your main meals to ease tummy discomfort and promote smooth digestion.

Important Cautions:

Stick to small amounts since turmeric can be quite strong and might upset sensitive stomachs if used too often.

Soothing Digestive Elixir with Apple Cider and Ginger

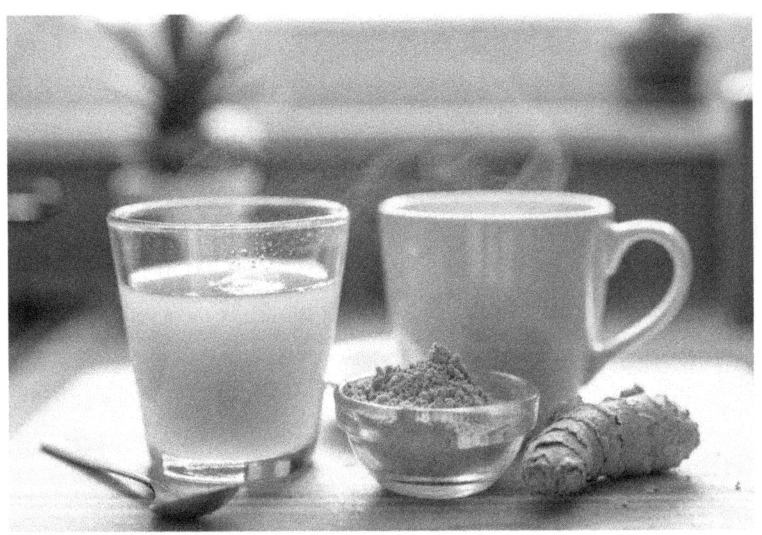

What You'll Need:

- 1 tablespoon of raw apple cider vinegar
- 1 teaspoon of ground ginger
- 1 cup of comfortably hot water

Steps to Prepare:

1. Pour the hot water into a mug.
2. Add the apple cider vinegar and ground ginger, then give it a good mix until everything blends together.
3. Sip it slowly while it's still warm.

Suggested Usage:

Enjoy this gentle blend first thing after waking up to help support smooth digestion and ease any puffiness in your belly throughout the day.

Important Cautions:

Skip this if your tummy tends to be easily upset or if you've got open sores in your stomach lining. Always check with a doctor if you're unsure about trying new home blends, especially if you have ongoing health concerns.

Homemade Spice and Citrus Dental Paste

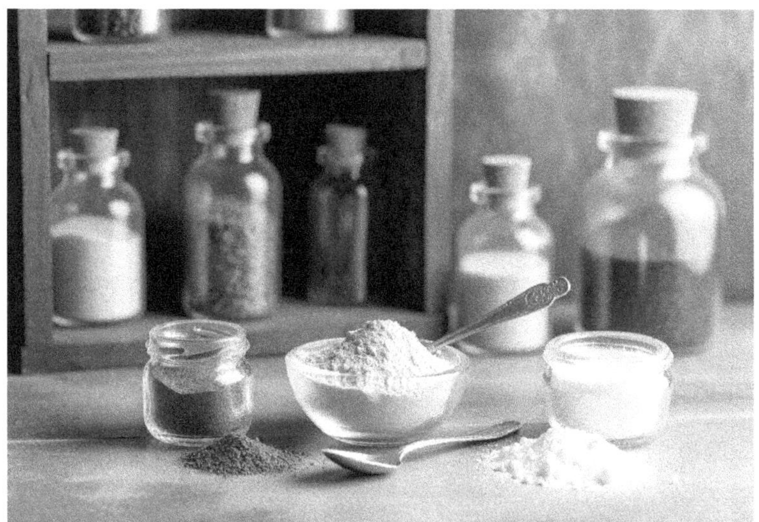

What You'll Need:

- 1/2 teaspoon of finely powdered cloves
- 1 tablespoon of powdered dried orange rind
- 1 tablespoon of baking soda
- 1 tablespoon of softened coconut oil

Steps to Prepare:

1. In a small dish, blend the powdered cloves, orange rind powder, and baking soda together until evenly combined.
2. Gradually add the coconut oil, stirring well to create a smooth, spreadable mixture.

Suggested Usage:

Apply a small amount to your toothbrush and brush your teeth gently each day to help maintain fresh breath and clean teeth.

Important Cautions:

Do not swallow the paste, as it is meant only for brushing and rinsing out.

Nettle and Rosemary Scalp Stimulating Rinse

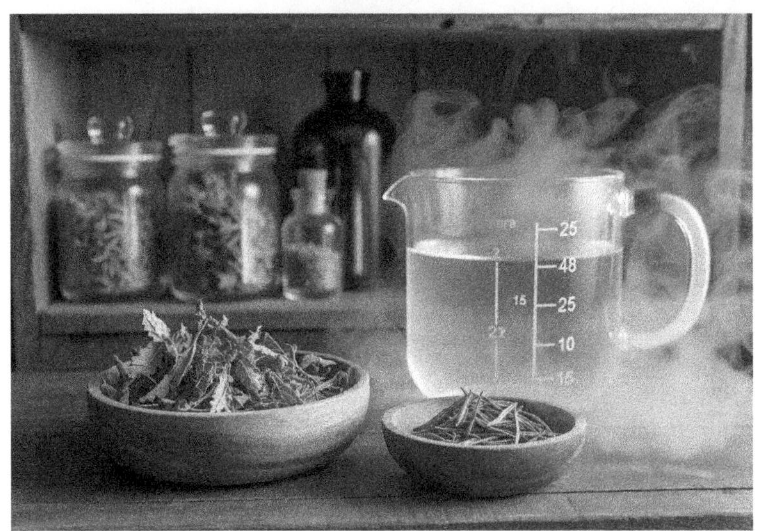

What You'll Need:

- 1 tablespoon dried nettle leaves
- 1 tablespoon dried rosemary leaves
- 2 cups freshly boiled water

Steps to Prepare:

1. Put the nettle and rosemary into a heat-safe bowl or jar.
2. Pour the hot water over the herbs and let them soak for 20 minutes.
3. Pour the liquid through a fine strainer to remove the plant bits.
4. Wait until it's cool enough to touch comfortably, then pour it over clean, washed hair as the last step in your routine.

Suggested Usage:

Apply this rinse 2-3 times each week to help support fuller, more vibrant hair over time.

Important Cautions:

Do not use it if your scalp tends to get irritated easily, as it could cause discomfort.

Citrus Root Energizer Brew

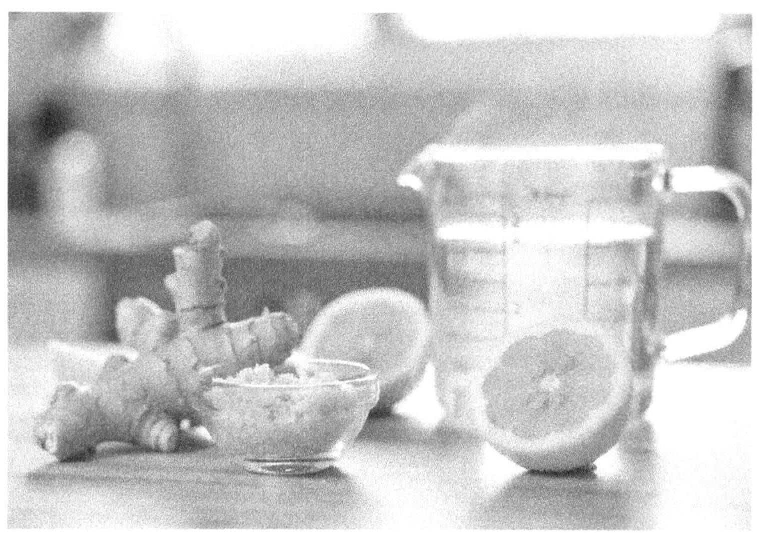

What You'll Need:

- 2 teaspoons finely chopped fresh ginger root
- Fresh squeeze from half a large lemon
- 8 ounces of boiling water

Steps to Prepare:

1. Place the chopped ginger in a mug and pour the boiling water over it.
2. Let it sit covered for about 7 minutes to draw out the flavors.
3. Filter out the ginger pieces, then stir in the lemon squeeze for a zesty kick.

Suggested Usage:

Sip this warm drink first thing each day to potentially aid your body's energy-burning rhythm and promote a sense of vitality.

Important Cautions:

Skip this if you often experience acid reflux or stomach discomfort, as the citrus might irritate sensitive digestion.

Peppermint and Tea Tree Congestion Clearing Inhalation

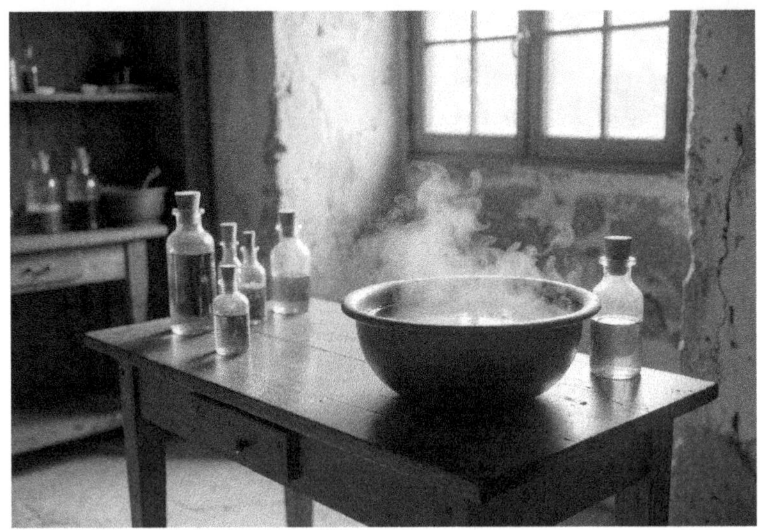

What You'll Need:

- 4 drops peppermint essential oil
- 1 drop tea tree essential oil
- A large basin filled with steaming water

Steps to Prepare:

1. Pour the steaming water into the basin.
2. Carefully mix in the essential oils.

Suggested Usage:

Lean over the basin, drape a cloth over your head to keep the vapors contained, and breathe deeply for about 12 minutes.

Important Cautions:

Skip this if you have sensitivity to any plant-based scents or oils.

Gentle Root and Citrus Cleansing Brew

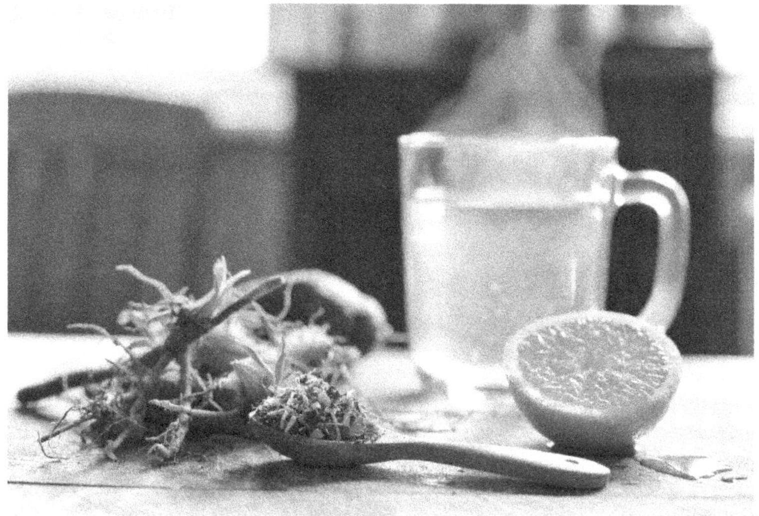

What You'll Need:

- 1 spoonful of chopped dried roots from the dandelion plant
- Fresh squeeze from half a small citrus fruit (about 1 spoonful of juice)
- 8 ounces of hot, just-boiled water

Steps to Prepare:

1. Place the dandelion roots in a mug and pour the hot water over them. Let it sit covered for about 15 minutes to draw out the natural essences.
2. Stir in the citrus juice, then pour through a fine mesh to remove any bits.

Suggested Usage:

Sip this warm beverage once or twice weekly to help support your body's natural cleaning processes, especially for gentle liver support.

Important Cautions:

Skip this if you're expecting a baby or nursing, as it might not be suitable during those times. Always check with a doctor if you have health concerns.

Revitalizing Facial Blend for Smooth Radiance

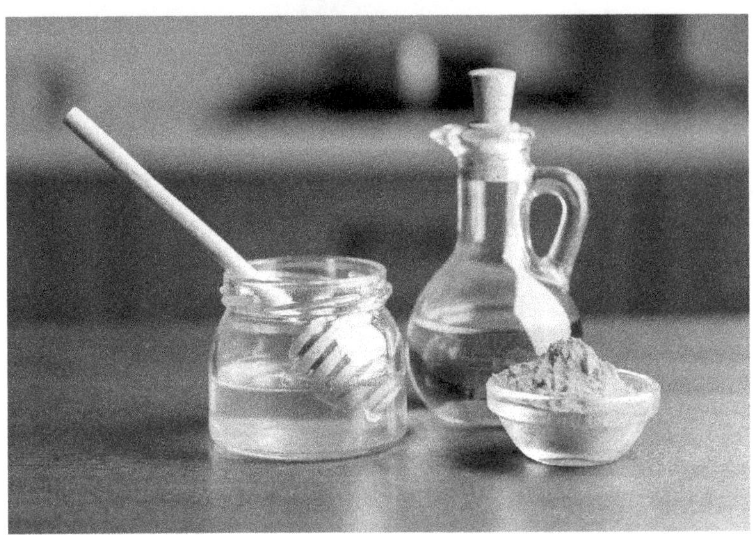

What You'll Need:

- 1 tablespoon natural honey
- 1 tablespoon extra virgin olive oil
- 1 teaspoon ground turmeric

Steps to Prepare:

1. Combine the honey, olive oil, and turmeric in a small dish.
2. Stir thoroughly until the mixture becomes smooth and even.

Suggested Usage:

Gently spread the blend over your clean face, then relax for around 20 minutes before washing it off with warm water. Try this routine weekly to help nourish your skin for a softer, more vibrant appearance.

Important Cautions:

Always apply a tiny bit to a small area of skin first, like your inner arm, and wait 24 hours to check for any signs of irritation or sensitivity.

Soothing Leaf Mix for Skin Blemishes

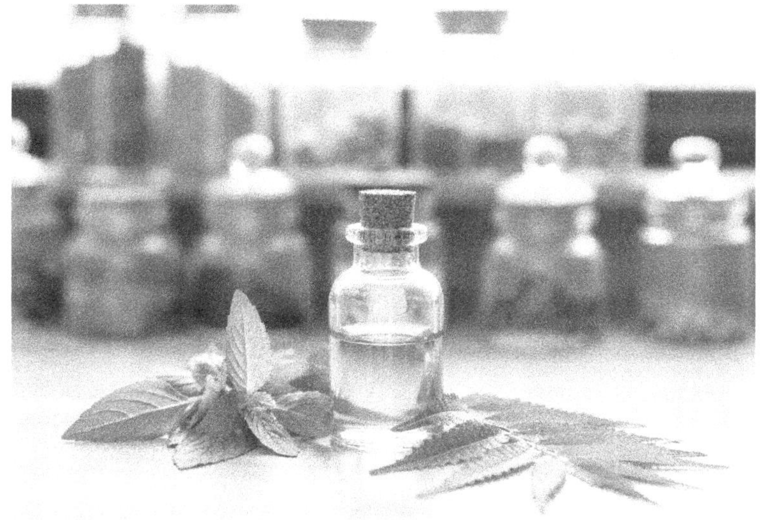

What You'll Need:

- A handful of fresh holy basil leaves (about 4-6)
- A handful of fresh neem leaves (about 4-6)
- 1 teaspoon of clean water

Steps to Prepare:

1. Crush the holy basil and neem leaves with the water using a mortar and pestle or blender until you get a smooth blend.
2. Spread the mixture gently on the spots where you have breakouts.

Suggested Usage:

Keep it on your skin for around 10-20 minutes, then wash away with cool water.

Important Cautions:

Avoid applying this if your skin has any cuts or open wounds.

Soothing Herb-Infused Soak for Unwinding

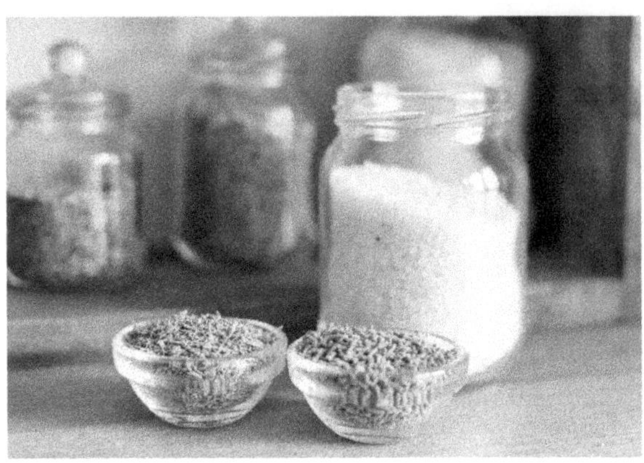

What You'll Need:

- 2 teaspoons of dried thyme leaves
- 2 teaspoons of dried lavender buds
- 3/4 cup of magnesium-rich bath salts (like Epsom)

Steps to Prepare:

1. Fill your tub with warm water to a comfortable level.
2. Sprinkle the thyme leaves, lavender buds, and bath salts directly into the water as it runs, stirring gently to help them disperse.
3. Allow the mixture to steep in the water for a few minutes before getting in.

Suggested Usage:

Enjoy this soak when you need to ease tight muscles or melt away daily tension. Aim for 15 to 25 minutes in the tub, perhaps in the evening to promote better rest.

Important Cautions:

Skip this if you know you're sensitive to lavender or thyme. Always do a small skin patch test first by placing a bit of the wet herbs on your arm and waiting 24 hours to check for any reaction. Consult a doctor if you're pregnant or have skin conditions.

Spicy Honey Soother for Sniffles

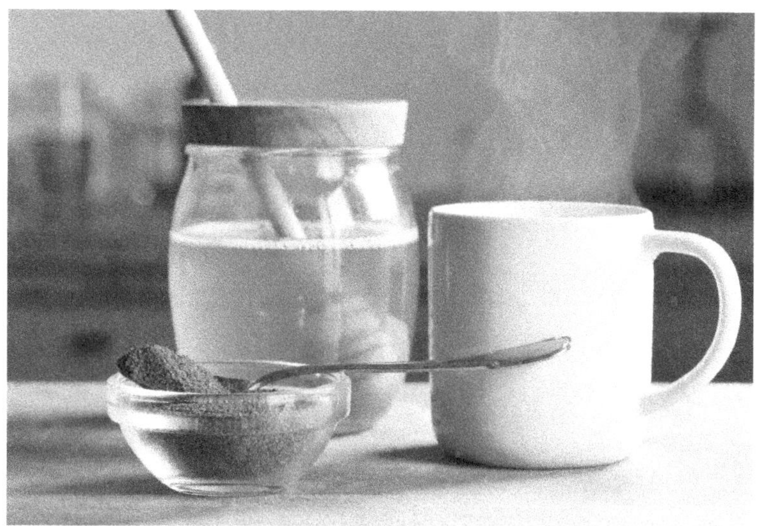

What You'll Need:

- A pinch (about 1/4 teaspoon) of ground red pepper
- 1 generous spoonful of natural honey
- Half a cup of comfortably hot water

Steps to Prepare:

1. Pour the hot water into a mug.
2. Add the ground red pepper and honey, then mix vigorously until everything blends smoothly.
3. Sip it right away while it's still warm.

Suggested Usage:

Take this drink up to two times daily when you're dealing with a stuffy nose or seasonal bug.

Important Cautions:

Skip this if your tummy tends to get upset easily, as the spice might irritate it. Always check with a doctor if symptoms persist.

Evergreen Twig and Spice Infusion for Breathing Support

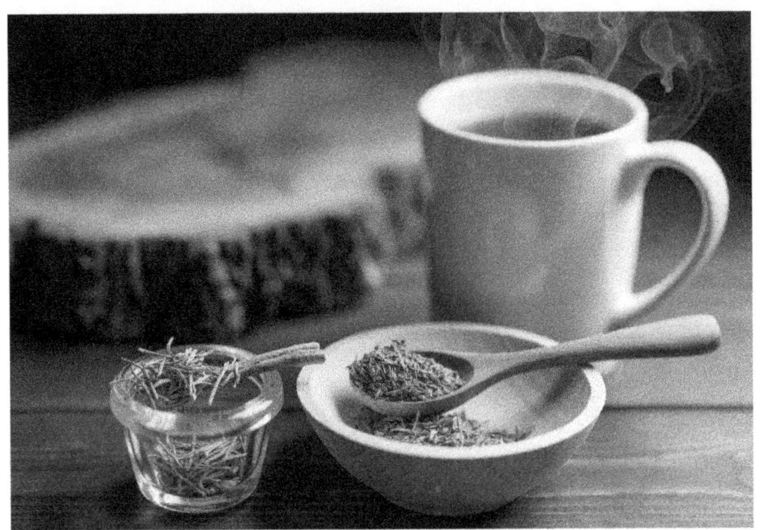

What You'll Need:

- A small bunch of dried evergreen needles (about a spoonful)
- A bit of fresh root spice, finely chopped (around half a spoonful)
- One mug of hot water

Steps to Prepare:

1. Place the evergreen needles and chopped root spice into a cup.
2. Pour the hot water over them and let it sit covered for about 15 minutes to draw out the flavors.
3. Filter out the solids and sip the warm liquid.

Suggested Usage:

Enjoy one cup each day to help ease breathing discomfort.

Important Cautions:

Skip this if you're expecting a baby.

Soothing Herbal Tea for Stomach Relief

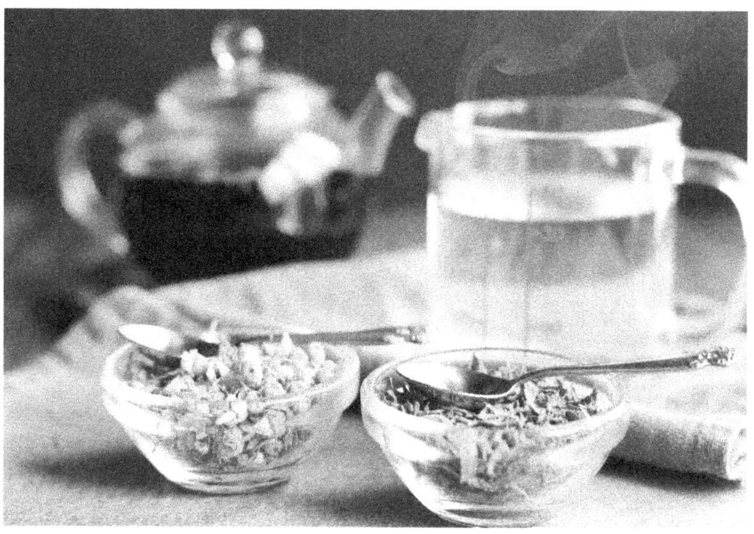

What You'll Need:

- 2 teaspoons of dried chamomile flowers
- 2 teaspoons of dried peppermint leaves
- 8 ounces of boiling water

Steps to Prepare:

1. Place the chamomile flowers and peppermint leaves into a mug or teapot.
2. Pour the boiling water over the herbs and let them sit covered for 7-10 minutes to release their natural essences.
3. Filter out the plant material using a fine mesh strainer, then enjoy the warm liquid.

Suggested Usage:

Sip this tea slowly right after eating to help calm your tummy and support smooth digestion.

Important Cautions:

Do not use it if you have known sensitivities to plants in the daisy family, such as ragweed, as it could cause a reaction. Consult a doctor if you are pregnant or have ongoing health issues.

Smooth Skin Elixir with Almond and Vitamin E

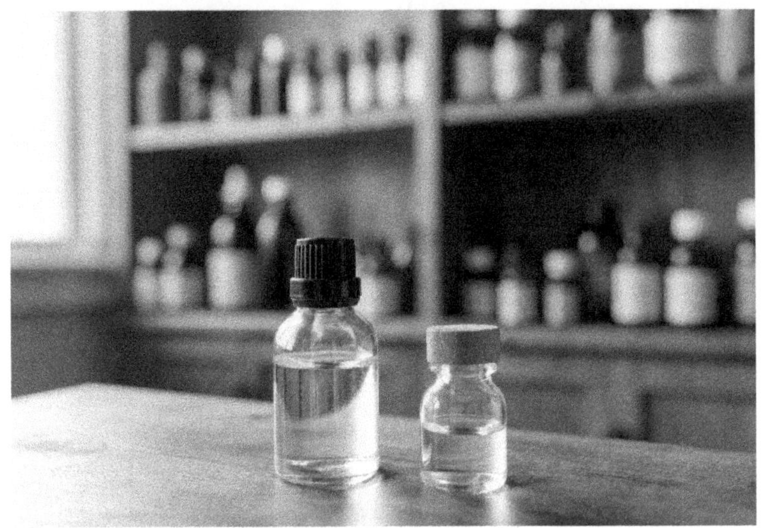

What You'll Need:

- 1 tablespoon sweet almond oil
- 1 teaspoon vitamin E oil

Steps to Prepare:

1. Pour the sweet almond oil into a clean, small glass jar.
2. Add the vitamin E oil and stir well with a clean spoon until fully combined.

Suggested Usage:

Gently massage a couple of drops onto clean skin each evening to help soften fine lines over time.

Important Cautions:

Skip this if you have allergies to nuts, as it may cause skin irritation. Always test a small patch on your arm first.

Natural Oat Polish with Honey and Citrus

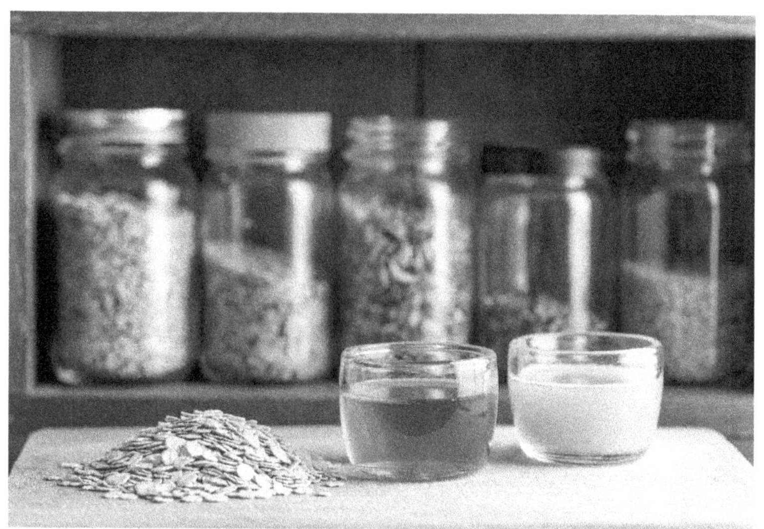

What You'll Need:

- 2 tablespoons of rolled oats
- 1 tablespoon of pure honey
- 1 teaspoon of fresh lemon juice

Steps to Prepare:

1. Use a blender or food processor to turn the oats into a smooth, powdery texture.
2. Combine the powdered oats with the honey and lemon juice in a small bowl, stirring until it becomes a thick, spreadable mixture.
3. Apply the blend to your face using light, swirling movements to buff away dullness.

Suggested Usage:

Apply this polish about once every seven days to refresh and add glow to your complexion.

Important Cautions:

Always test a small amount on your inner arm first to check for any reaction to the citrus element.

Soothing Carrot and Spice Face Treatment

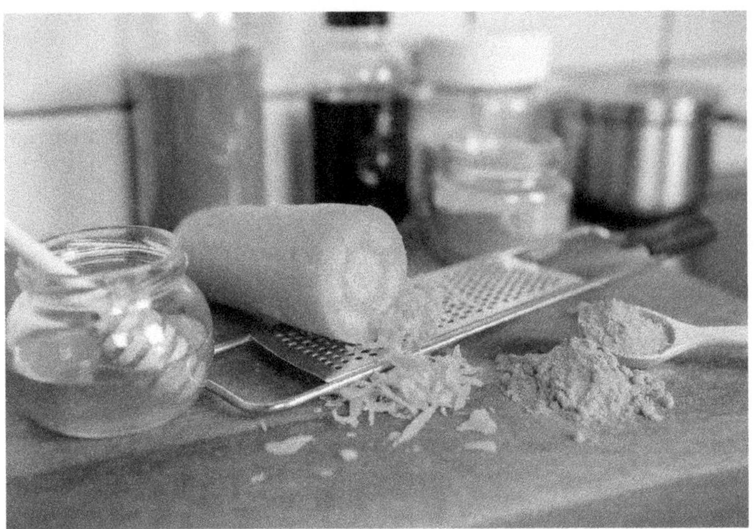

What You'll Need:

- 1 small carrot, grated fresh
- 1 teaspoon ground turmeric
- 1 tablespoon honey

Steps to Prepare:

1. Stir together the grated carrot, ground turmeric, and honey until it forms a smooth mix.
2. Spread the mix evenly over your clean face and let it sit for 10-15 minutes before rinsing off with cool water.

Suggested Usage:

Apply this gentle treatment once every seven days to help calm red or puffy skin and give your face a fresh, even look.

Important Cautions:

Stay away from this if you know you're sensitive to turmeric, as it might cause skin irritation.

Herbal Oil Blend for Promoting Hair Vitality

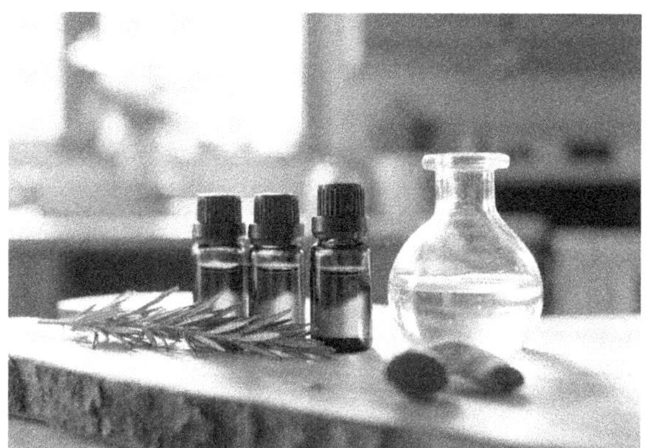

What You'll Need:

- 3 drops of rosemary essential oil
- 2 drops of cinnamon essential oil
- 2 tablespoons of jojoba oil (as a gentle base)

Steps to Prepare:

1. In a small dish, combine the rosemary and cinnamon essential oils with the jojoba oil.
2. Stir gently until everything is well blended.
3. For better absorption, warm the mixture slightly by placing the dish in a bowl of hot water for a minute or two.

Suggested Usage:

Rub the blend into your scalp using your fingertips in circular motions. Let it soak in for about 45 minutes, then rinse thoroughly with a mild cleanser. Try this every seven days to help nourish your hair roots and support natural growth.

Important Cautions:

Skip this if you're expecting a baby or have a known sensitivity to cinnamon, as it might cause irritation. Always do a small skin test first on your arm to check for any reaction.

Soothing Aloe and Mint Foot Rub

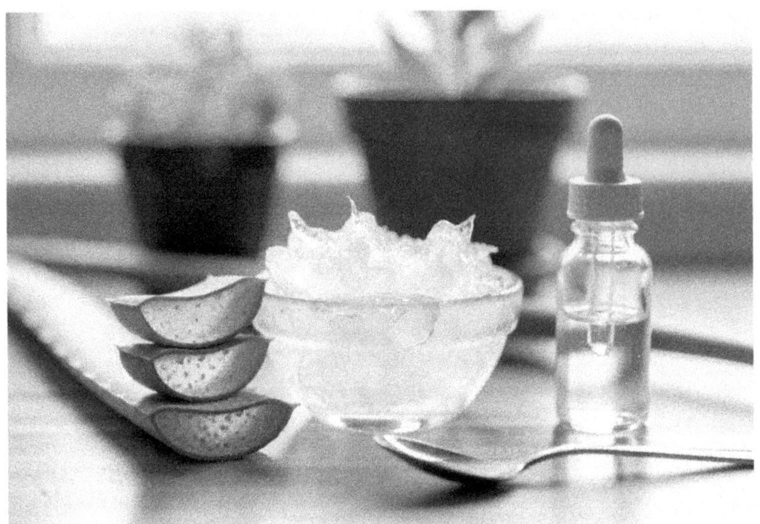

What You'll Need:

- 3 tablespoons of aloe vera gel from the plant
- 1 teaspoon of melted coconut oil
- 4 drops of peppermint oil for scent

Steps to Prepare:

1. Blend the aloe gel and coconut oil in a small bowl until smooth.
2. Stir in the peppermint oil to combine everything well.

Suggested Usage:

Rub a small amount onto clean feet with light circular motions, then rinse off after a few minutes. Try this routine a few times each week to help keep your feet feeling fresh and smooth.

Important Cautions:

Do not use it if your skin tends to react easily to new products. Always test a tiny bit on your arm first.

Natural Fungus-Fighting Mix Using Clove and Olive

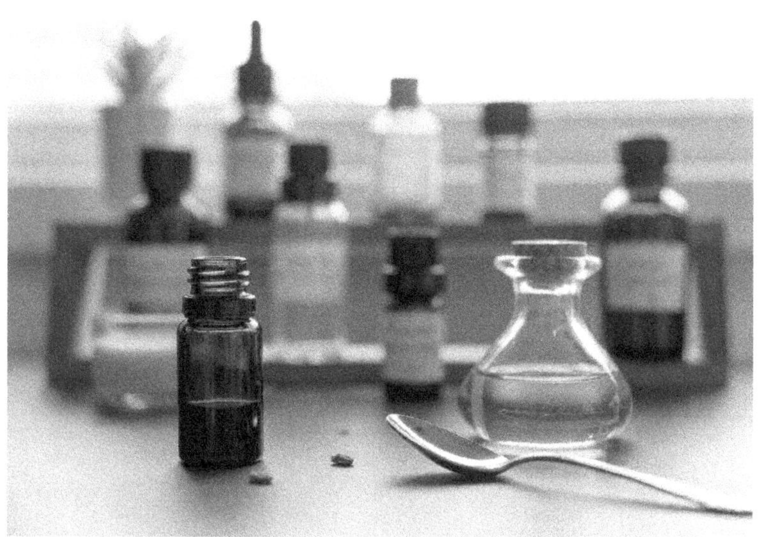

What You'll Need:

- 2 drops of clove essential oil
- 1 tablespoon of olive oil

Steps to Prepare:

1. Blend the clove essential oil thoroughly into the olive oil.
2. Gently spread the mixture onto areas affected by fungus, for example, on toes or feet prone to itchiness from conditions like athlete's foot.

Suggested Usage:

Dab it on the troubled spots two to three times a day, continuing until the irritation eases and clears up.

Important Cautions:

Before full use, apply a tiny amount to a small patch of skin to make sure there's no redness or discomfort.

Soothing Herbal Balm for Calming Redness

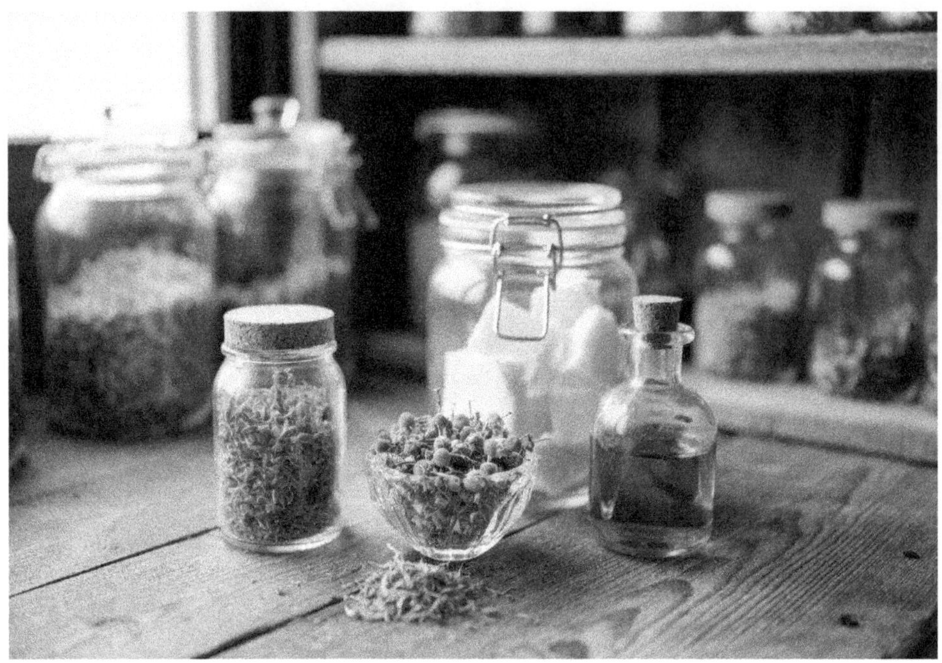

What You'll Need:

- 1 spoonful of dried marigold petals (also known as calendula)
- 1 spoonful of dried German chamomile blossoms
- 2 spoonfuls of cocoa butter
- Enough olive oil to cover the herbs (about 4 spoonfuls)

Steps to Prepare:

1. Place the marigold petals and chamomile blossoms in a small jar, then pour in the olive oil until the herbs are fully submerged. Let this sit in a warm spot, like near a window with sunlight, for about 2 hours to draw out the gentle properties.
2. Pour the mixture through a fine cloth or strainer to remove the plant bits, keeping only the flavored oil.
3. Gently warm the cocoa butter in a bowl over hot water until it softens, then stir in the flavored oil until everything blends smoothly into a creamy paste. Let it cool and firm up before storing in a clean container.

Suggested Usage:

Gently rub a small amount onto areas of dry, itchy, or sun-exposed skin as needed for relief. It's great for everyday comfort after time outdoors.

Important Cautions:

Do not use on open cuts or wounds. Always test a tiny patch on your arm first to check for any skin reaction, and stop if it feels uncomfortable. Keep away from eyes and consult a doctor if issues persist.

Soothing Herbal Under-Eye Blend

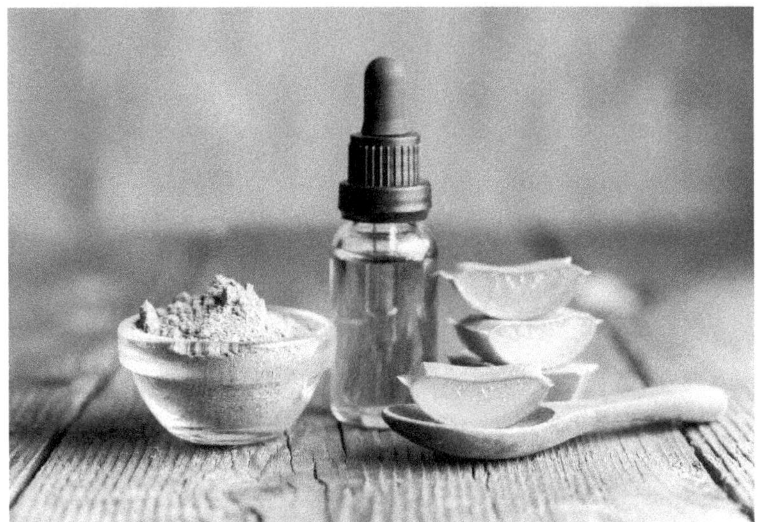

What You'll Need:

- 2 teaspoons finely ground licorice root
- ½ teaspoon concentrated green tea liquid
- 2 teaspoons fresh aloe vera jelly

Steps to Prepare:

1. Blend the ground licorice root with the green tea liquid until it forms a light mixture.
2. Stir in the aloe vera jelly gradually to create an even, spreadable consistency.
3. Store in a small, clean container if not using right away.

Suggested Usage:

Dab a tiny amount onto the skin beneath and around your eyes each evening, allowing it to absorb while you rest, to help fade tired-looking areas and ease morning swell.

Important Cautions:

Keep the blend away from direct eye contact to prevent irritation. If any discomfort occurs, rinse with cool water and stop use.

Refreshing Cucumber Blend for Moisturized Skin

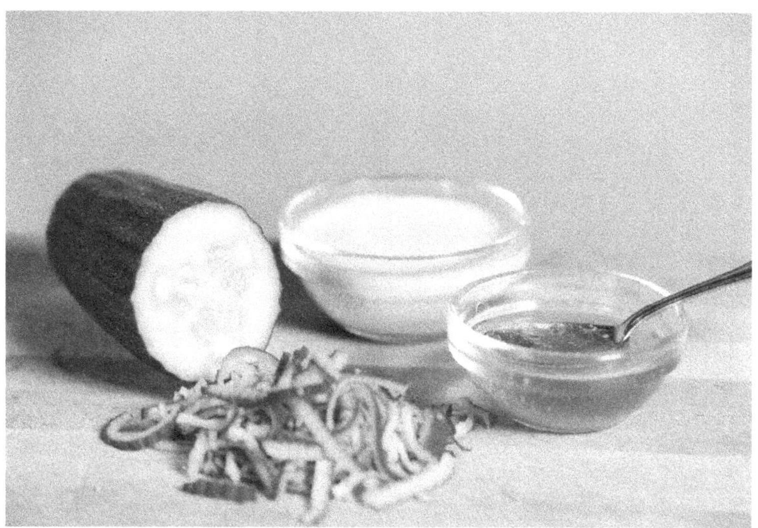

What You'll Need:

- Half a fresh cucumber, finely shredded
- Two tablespoons of creamy coconut liquid
- One tablespoon of natural sweetener like honey

Steps to Prepare:

1. Shred the cucumber into small pieces and combine it with the coconut liquid and sweetener in a bowl.
2. Stir everything together until it forms a smooth paste.
3. Spread the mixture evenly over your clean face and let it sit for about 15 to 20 minutes before rinsing off with cool water.

Suggested Usage:

Use this blend a couple of times each week to help add moisture and revive tired, dry skin.

Important Cautions:

Skip this if you have any sensitivity to coconut products, and always test a small area of skin first to check for reactions.

Berry Boost Blend for Sniffles and Shivers

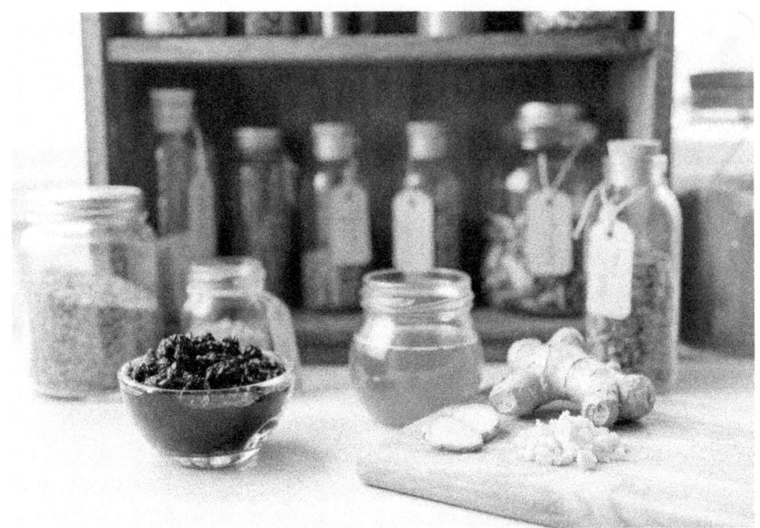

What You'll Need:

- 1/4 cup elderberry concentrate
- 1 tablespoon peeled and finely chopped ginger root
- 1 tablespoon raw honey

Steps to Prepare:

1. Gather everything in a clean glass container.
2. Blend thoroughly until smooth, then it's ready to use right away.

Suggested Usage:

Spoon out 1 tablespoon a couple of times daily, or up to three doses, to help ease discomfort from seasonal bugs.

Important Cautions:

Skip this for infants less than a year old due to honey concerns.

Soothing Fennel and Peppermint Blend for Tummy Relief

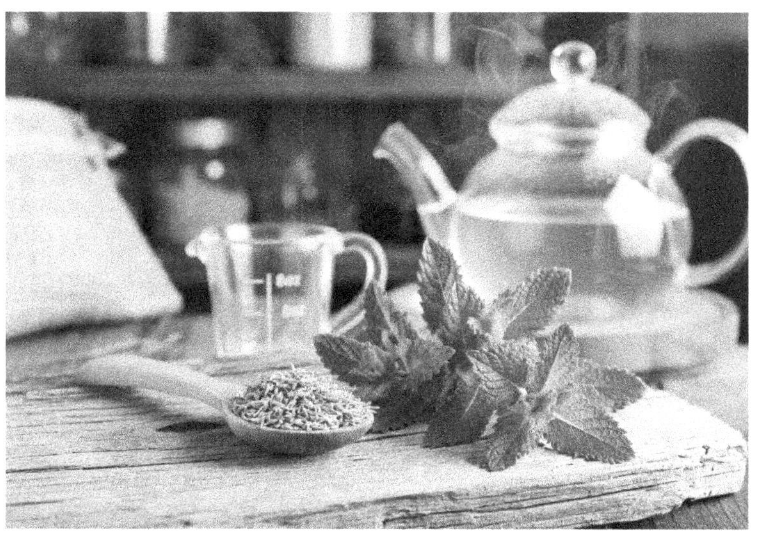

What You'll Need:

- 1 small spoonful of dried fennel seeds
- A generous pinch of fresh peppermint leaves
- 8 ounces of boiling water

Steps to Prepare:

1. Add the fennel seeds and peppermint leaves to a mug.
2. Pour the boiling water over the mixture.
3. Allow it to sit covered for about 7 minutes to draw out the flavors.
4. Pour through a sieve to remove the solids, then sip while warm.

Suggested Usage:

Enjoy a cup right after eating to help calm your stomach and support smooth digestion.

Important Cautions:

Skip this if you're expecting a baby or nursing, as it might not be suitable.

Daily Defense Tonic with Nigella Oil and Garlic

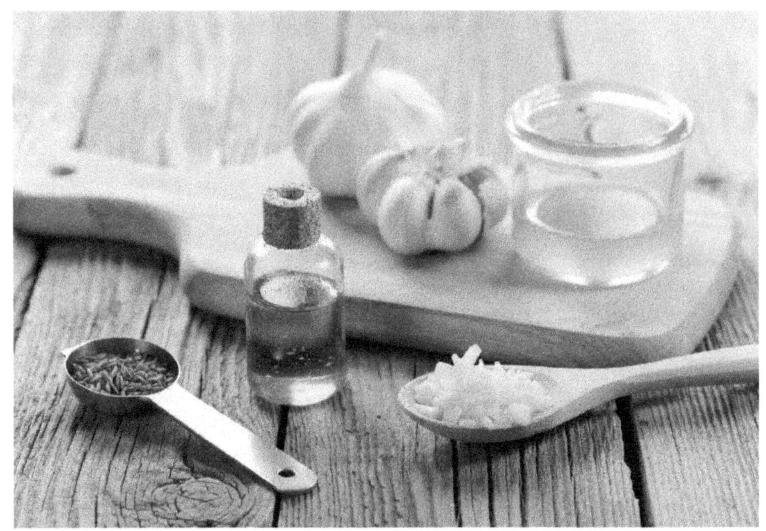

What You'll Need:

- 1 tablespoon nigella seed oil
- 2 fresh garlic bulbs, finely chopped
- 1 teaspoon natural sweetener like honey

Steps to Prepare:

1. Combine the nigella seed oil and chopped garlic in a small container.
2. Add the honey and stir everything together until smooth.

Suggested Usage:

Spoon out a small amount first thing each day to help your body stay strong against common bugs.

Important Cautions:

Skip this if you react badly to garlic or nigella products. Talk to a healthcare provider before starting, especially with any health conditions.

Golden Spice and Sweetener Spot Remedy

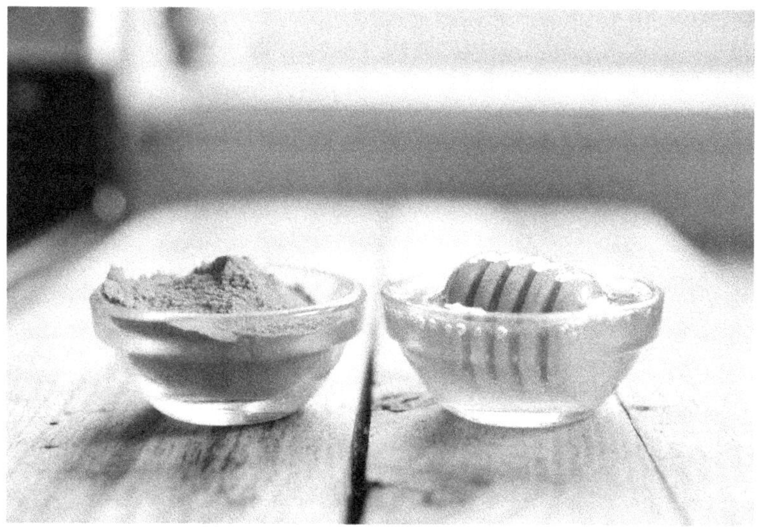

What You'll Need:

- 1 small spoonful of ground turmeric
- 2 small spoonfuls of raw honey

Steps to Prepare:

1. Stir the ground turmeric into the raw honey until you get a thick, even blend.
2. Spread the mixture gently onto the spots where breakouts appear, and let it sit for about a quarter of an hour before rinsing off with warm water.

Suggested Usage:

Use this blend once a day to help calm redness and clear up pimples over time.

Important Cautions:

This may not suit very delicate skin, so try a small test spot on your arm first to check for any irritation.

Relaxing Herb Blend for Restful Evenings

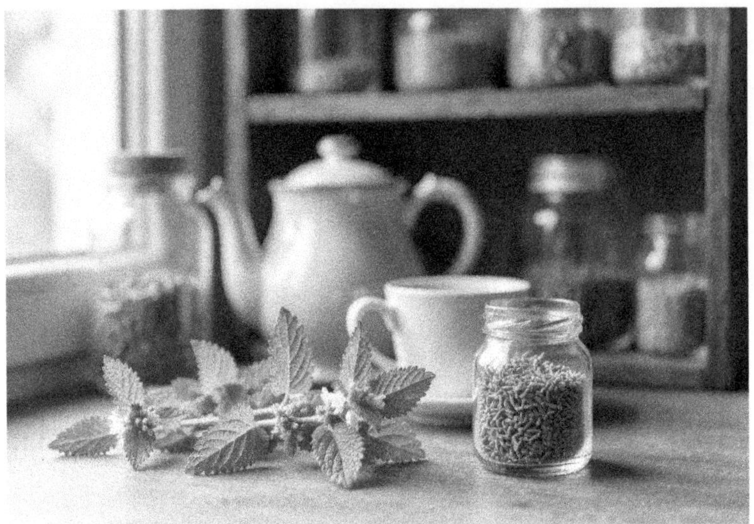

What You'll Need:

- A small handful of fresh lemon balm sprigs (about 2 teaspoons chopped)
- 1 teaspoon of lavender buds (dried works best)
- 8 ounces of boiling water

Steps to Prepare:

1. Place the lemon balm and lavender into a mug or teapot.
2. Pour the boiling water over the herbs and cover to keep the aromas in.
3. Let it sit for around 8-12 minutes to draw out the calming essences.
4. Filter out the plant bits using a strainer, then sip slowly.

Suggested Usage:

Enjoy this warm drink about an hour before you head to bed each evening to help unwind and encourage deeper rest.

Important Cautions:

Skip this if you're expecting a baby or nursing, as it might not be suitable. Always check with a doctor if you have health concerns.

Energizing Root Infusion

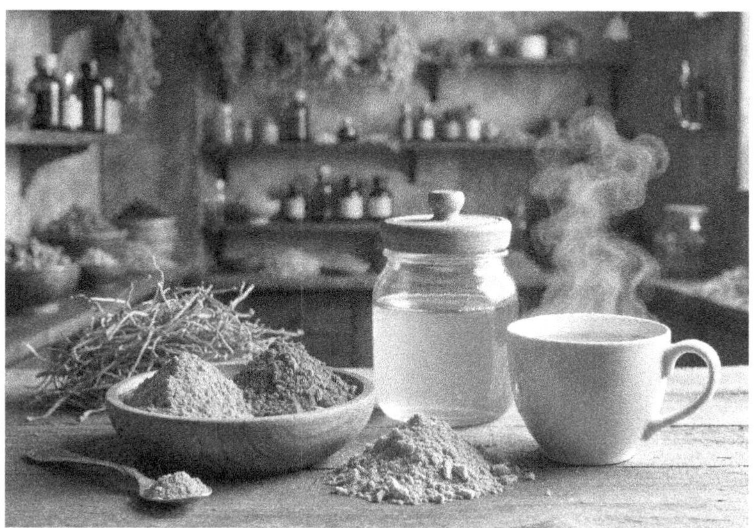

What You'll Need:

- 1/2 teaspoon ashwagandha root powder
- 1/2 teaspoon ginseng root powder
- 2 teaspoons natural honey
- 8 ounces hot water

Steps to Prepare:

1. Add the ashwagandha and ginseng powders to a large mug.
2. Pour the hot water over the powders and let them steep for about 5 minutes.
3. Stir in the honey until it fully dissolves.

Suggested Usage:

Sip this gently upon waking to help keep your stamina steady from morning to evening.

Important Cautions:

Check with a healthcare professional before trying this if you deal with raised blood pressure or take any prescribed drugs.

Soothing Balm for Red, Swollen Skin

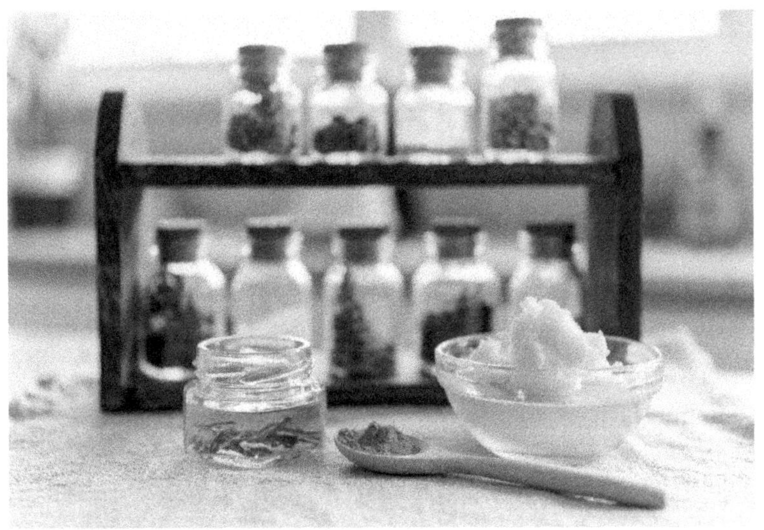

What You'll Need:

- 1 tablespoon of neem extract oil
- 1 teaspoon of ground turmeric root
- 2 tablespoons of melted shea butter

Steps to Prepare:

1. Combine the neem extract oil with the ground turmeric root in a small bowl.
2. Stir in the melted shea butter until everything blends into a smooth paste.
3. Let the mixture cool and thicken slightly before use.

Suggested Usage:

Gently spread a thin layer on affected spots and leave it on for about 10-15 minutes, then rinse off. Try this a couple of times per week to help ease discomfort from swelling.

Important Cautions:

Skip this if you have sensitivity to shea products or any of the components. Test on a small skin patch first to check for reactions, and consult a doctor if swelling persists.

Soothing Red Pepper Honey Drink for Throat Ease

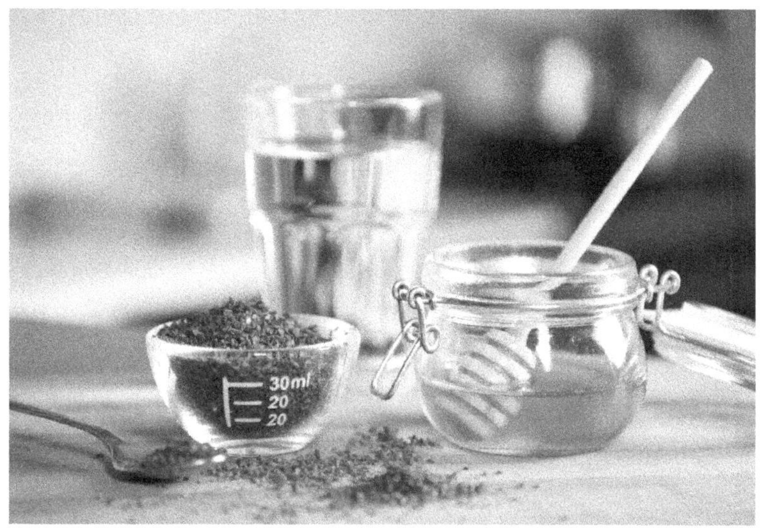

What You'll Need:

- 1/4 teaspoon ground red chili pepper
- 1 tablespoon pure honey
- 1/2 cup heated water

Steps to Prepare:

1. Add the chili pepper and honey to a cup.
2. Pour the heated water over them and blend until smooth.
3. Drink it in small amounts over time.

Suggested Usage:

Enjoy one or two servings each day to help calm throat irritation.

Important Cautions:

Steer clear if hot spices cause discomfort or reactions.

Soothing Spice Brew for Digestion

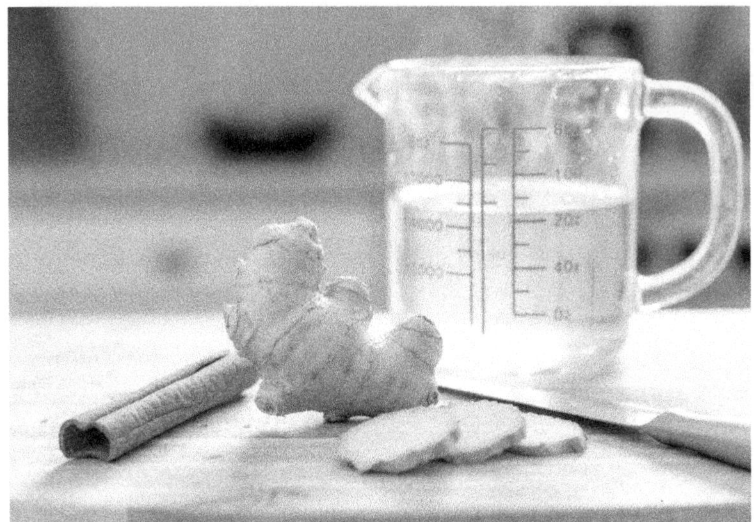

What You'll Need:

- A small knob of fresh ginger root (about thumb-sized), thinly cut
- One whole cinnamon bark piece
- 8 ounces of boiling water

Steps to Prepare:

1. Place the cut ginger and cinnamon bark into a mug.
2. Pour the boiling water over them and let it sit covered for around 8-12 minutes to draw out the flavors.
3. Remove the solids with a fine mesh or spoon, then sip it hot.

Suggested Usage:

Enjoy a cup following your main meals to ease queasiness or tummy upset.

Important Cautions:

Skip this if you're expecting a baby or taking meds that thin the blood.

Coneflower Blossom Defense Brew

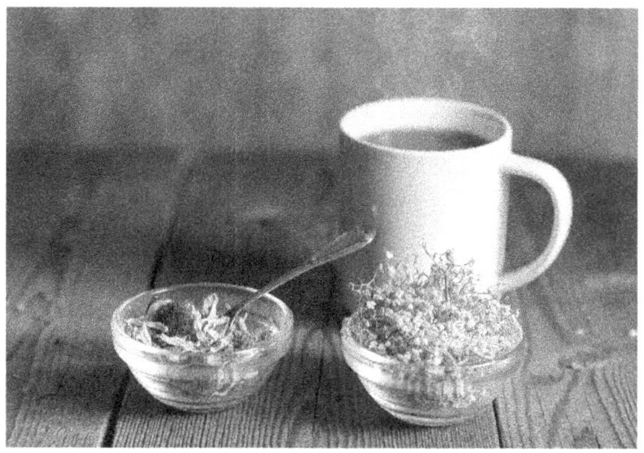

What You'll Need:

- A spoonful of dried coneflower petals
- A spoonful of dried elder blossoms
- One mug of boiling water

Steps to Prepare:

1. Place the coneflower petals and elder blossoms into a mug.
2. Pour the boiling water over them and let the mixture sit covered for around 7 minutes to draw out the natural essences.
3. Pour through a fine mesh to remove the plant bits, then sip while warm.

Suggested Usage:

Enjoy this gentle infusion a few times each week as part of your routine to help support your body's natural resistance during busy seasons or when feeling run down. For added flavor, stir in a dash of fresh lemon juice or a touch of raw honey after straining.

Important Cautions:

Steer clear of this if you know you're sensitive to flowers in the daisy group, as it might cause discomfort like itching or swelling. Always check with a healthcare provider if you're pregnant, nursing, or on medications.

Refreshing Beet and Carrot Cleanse Blend

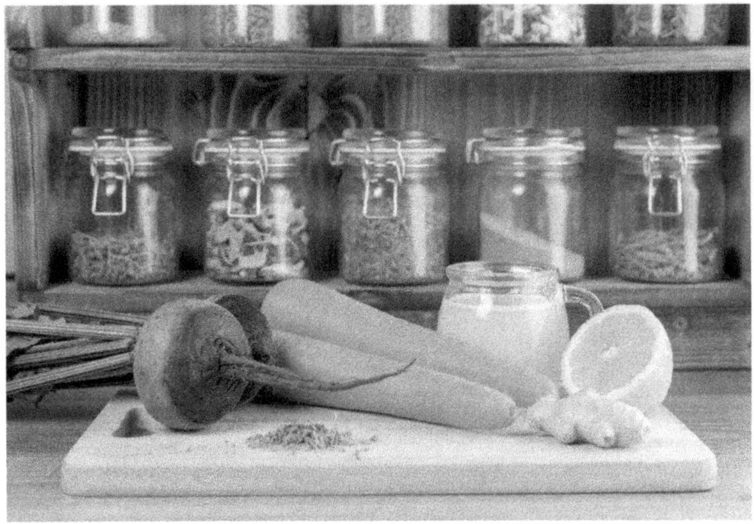

What You'll Need:

- One medium beet, with the outer skin taken off
- Two medium carrots, outer layer removed
- Fresh juice squeezed from half a lemon
- A small section of fresh ginger root, about the length of your thumb tip

Steps to Prepare:

1. Feed the beet, carrots, and ginger into a juicer to extract their liquids.
2. Add the lemon juice to the mixture, give it a good mix, and enjoy it right away.

Suggested Usage:

Sip this blend first thing in the day before eating anything to help support your body's natural cleansing process.

Important Cautions:

Steer clear of this if you're dealing with issues like stones in the kidneys.

Gentle Liver Support Brew with Dandelion and Ginger

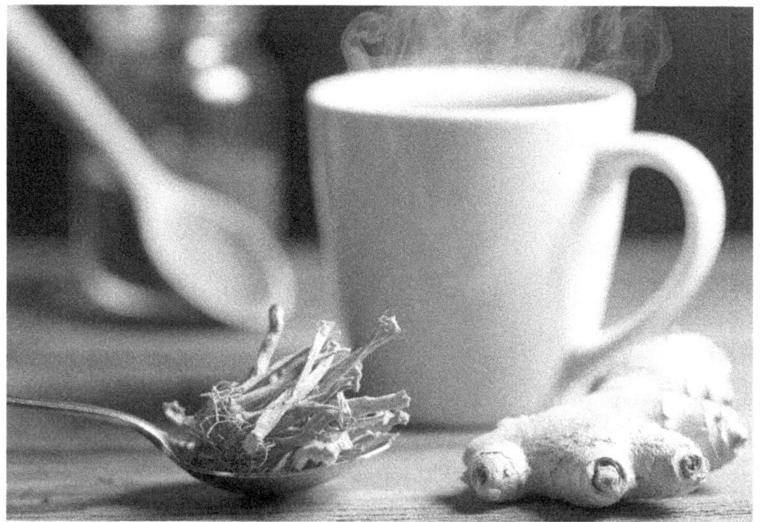

What You'll Need:

- A teaspoon of dried dandelion root
- A thin slice of fresh ginger root (roughly half an inch)
- One mug of boiling water

Steps to Prepare:

1. Add the dandelion root and ginger slice to a heat-safe mug.
2. Pour the boiling water over the items.
3. Cover the mug and allow the mixture to infuse for about 15 minutes.
4. Remove the solids by pouring through a fine mesh strainer, then sip the warm liquid.

Suggested Usage:

Enjoy this brew one or two times each week to help maintain healthy liver function.

Important Cautions:

If you have any ongoing liver concerns or take medications, check with a doctor before starting this.

Hibiscus and Rose Petal Skin Toner

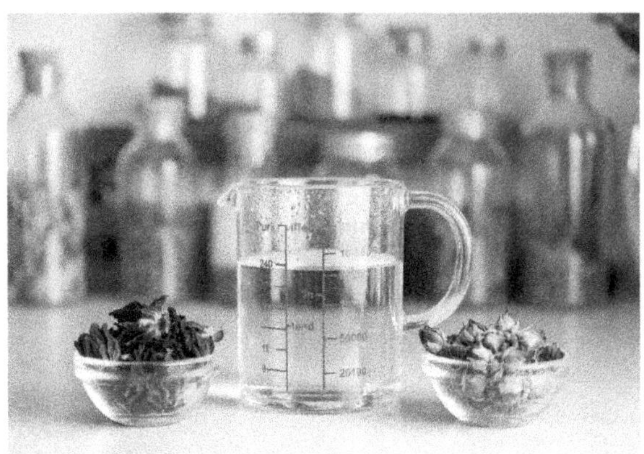

What You'll Need:

- 1 tablespoon of dried hibiscus blooms
- 1 tablespoon of dried rose buds
- 1 cup of purified water

Steps to Prepare:

1. Heat the water until it's just starting to steam, but not fully boiling, to keep the natural goodness intact.
2. Add the hibiscus blooms and rose buds to the hot water, cover, and let them soak for about 15 minutes.
3. Once cooled, pour through a fine mesh strainer to remove the plant pieces, then transfer the liquid to a clean glass jar for keeping.

Suggested Usage:

Dab a bit onto a soft cloth or cotton ball after washing your face, then gently swipe it over your skin to help brighten and refresh your look.

Important Cautions:

Don't use this if your skin tends to get easily irritated or if you know you're sensitive to these types of plants. Always do a small patch test first on your arm to check for any reaction.

Nutrient-Rich Leaf Mix for Healthier Tresses

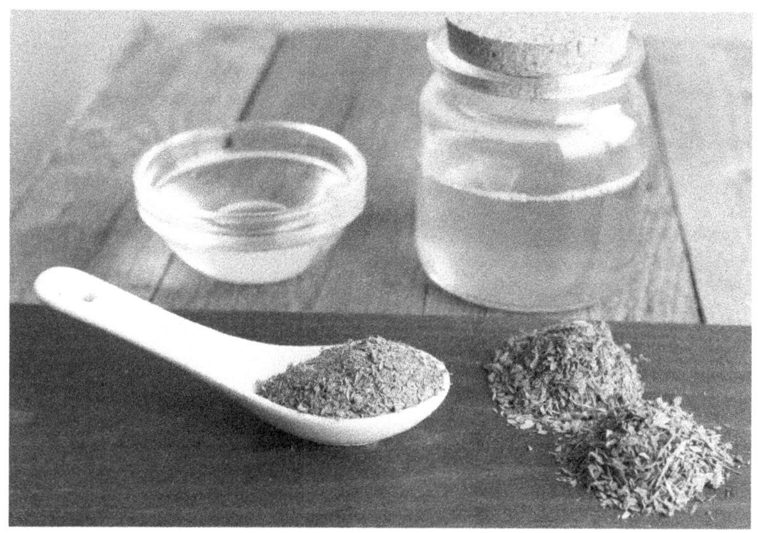

What You'll Need:

- 1 spoonful of finely ground moringa leaves
- 2 spoonfuls of natural honey
- 1 spoonful of coconut oil

Steps to Prepare:

1. Blend the ground moringa leaves with the honey and coconut oil until you get a creamy blend.
2. Gently massage the mixture onto your scalp and let it rest for about half an hour before rinsing off with lukewarm water.

Suggested Usage:

Try this treatment every seven days to help support stronger and fuller hair over time.

Important Cautions:

Do a small skin test on your arm first to make sure you don't have any irritation or sensitivity to the mix.

Soothing Herbal Oat Bath Blend

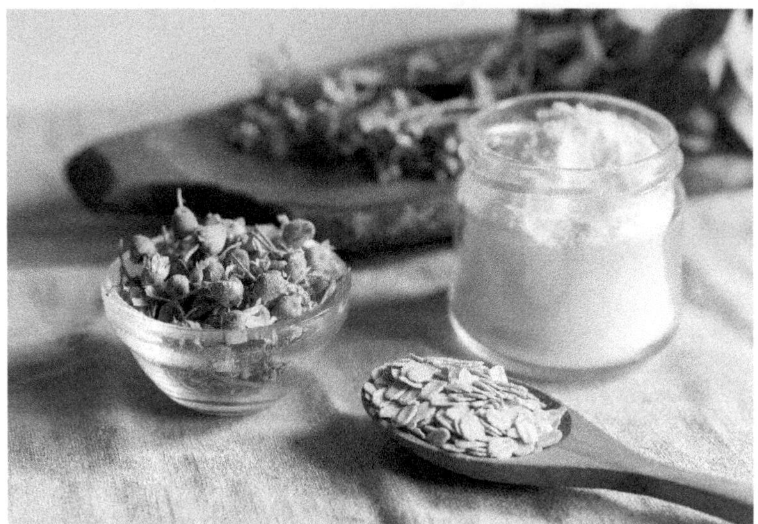

What You'll Need:

- 1/2 cup dried chamomile blossoms
- 1/2 cup rolled oats
- 1/4 cup baking soda

Steps to Prepare:

1. Combine the chamomile blossoms, rolled oats, and baking soda in a small cloth pouch or sock.
2. Secure the top tightly with a string or rubber band.

Suggested Usage:

Draw a warm tub of water, place the pouch under the running faucet to let the goodness infuse, and relax in the bath for 15-25 minutes to ease tension and soften your skin.

Important Cautions:

Skip this if you have a known sensitivity to chamomile.

Natural Blend for Combating Skin Fungus

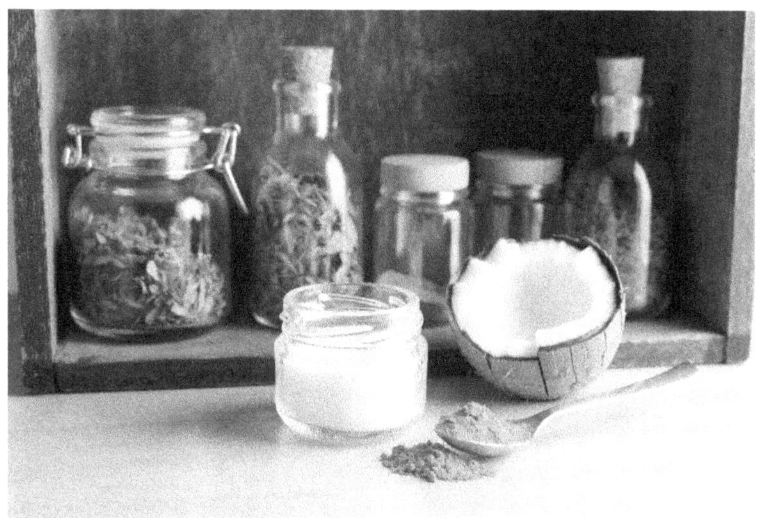

What You'll Need:

- 1 spoonful of virgin coconut oil
- A pinch (about 1/4 teaspoon) of ground turmeric

Steps to Prepare:

1. Gently warm the coconut oil in a small bowl until it's soft and easy to stir.
2. Sprinkle in the turmeric and blend thoroughly to create a uniform paste.

Suggested Usage:

Spread a thin layer on the troubled spots, let it sit for about 20 minutes, then rinse off. Repeat every other day to help manage minor fungal concerns on the skin.

Important Cautions:

Steer clear of applying near eyes or other delicate zones. This mixture might leave a temporary yellow tint on your skin or clothes, so use old towels if needed. Always test on a small patch first to check for any irritation.

Cooling Cucumber Aloe Facial Blend

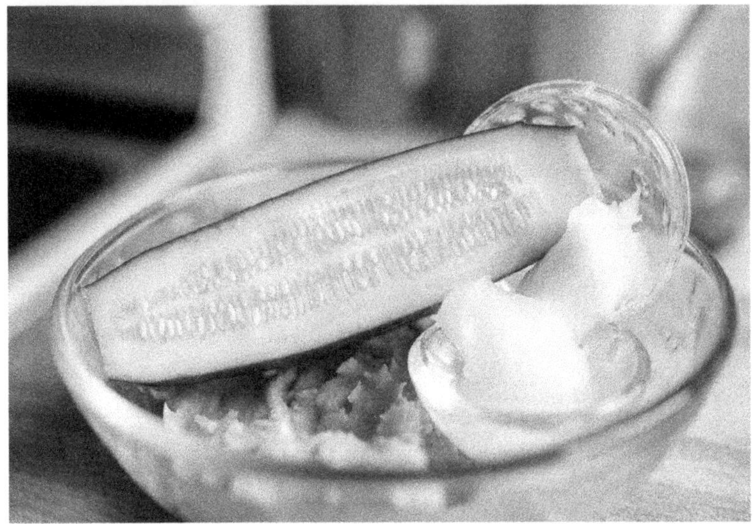

What You'll Need:

- Half a fresh cucumber, pureed into a smooth paste
- 2 tablespoons of fresh aloe vera gel (from the leaf or store-bought pure gel)

Steps to Prepare:

1. Cut the cucumber into chunks and puree it in a blender or food processor until it's completely smooth.
2. Scoop the puree into a small bowl and stir in the aloe vera gel until fully combined into a creamy mixture.

Suggested Usage:

Spread a thin layer over your clean face, avoiding the eyes, and relax for 15 minutes. Rinse off with cool water. This blend works well to refresh and moisten parched skin or ease discomfort from too much sun exposure.

Important Cautions:

Always try a small amount on your inner arm first to make sure your skin doesn't react badly. If you notice redness or itching, stop using it right away.

Refreshing Herb Citrus Purifier Drink

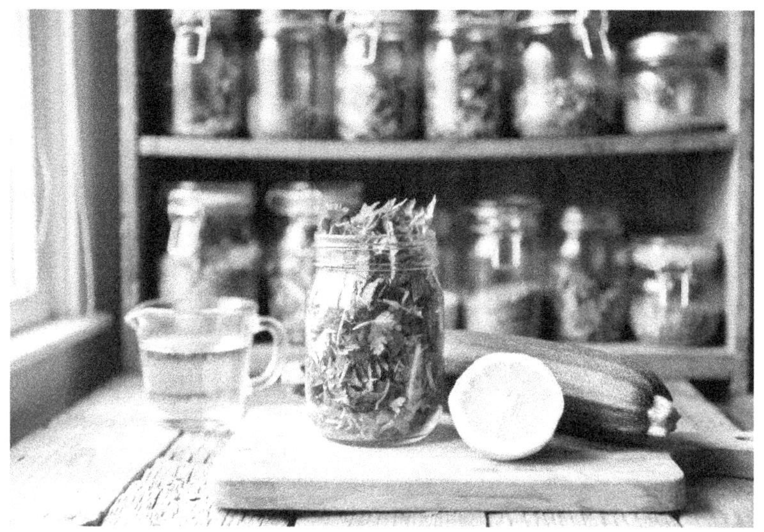

What You'll Need:

- 1 cup chopped fresh parsley
- Juice of 1/2 lemon
- 1/2 medium zucchini
- 1/2 cup filtered water

Steps to Prepare:

1. Rinse the parsley and zucchini under cool water.
2. Add everything to a blender and mix on high speed until it becomes a uniform liquid.

Suggested Usage:

Enjoy this beverage right after waking up to support your body's natural cleansing process.

Important Cautions:

Speak with a healthcare professional before trying if you are using any cleansing treatments or have liver concerns.

Natural Blend for Blemish Relief

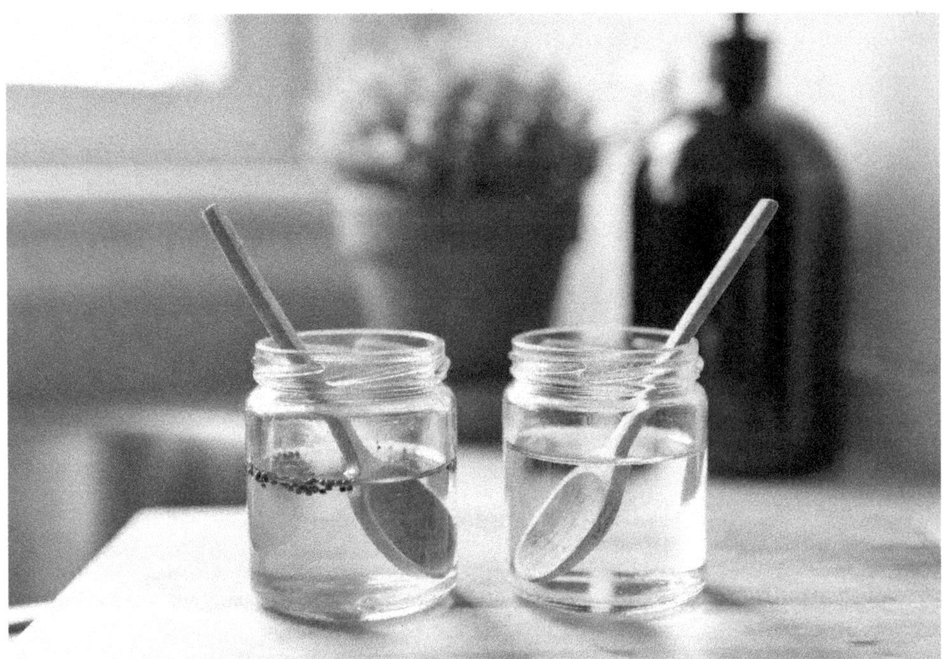

What You'll Need:

- One spoonful of oil from grape seeds
- One spoonful of jojoba plant oil

Steps to Prepare:

1. Pour both oils into a clean container.
2. Stir them gently until fully combined.

Suggested Usage:

Dab a small amount onto spots with pimples each evening before sleep.

Important Cautions:

Always try a tiny bit on your inner arm first to make sure your skin doesn't react badly before applying it often.

Saffron and Honey Eye Brightening Serum

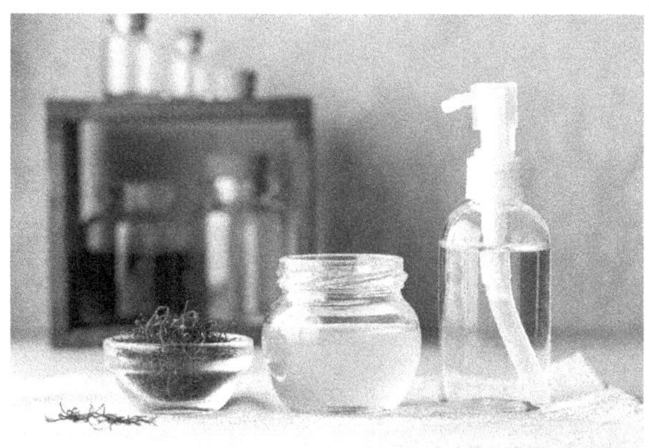

What You'll Need:

- ¼ teaspoon of saffron strands
- 1 tablespoon of pure honey
- 1 tablespoon of rose water

Steps to Prepare:

Place the saffron strands, honey, and rose water in a small, clean bowl. Stir everything together gently until the saffron releases its color and the ingredients form a smooth, golden mixture.

Suggested Usage:

Each night before bedtime, apply a thin layer of the blend gently around your eyes using clean fingertips. Regular use may help fade the look of dark circles and ease puffiness for brighter, refreshed eyes.

Important Cautions:

Always test a small amount on your inner forearm first and wait 24 hours to check for any redness or irritation, especially if you have sensitive skin. Do not get the mixture in your eyes. If irritation occurs, stop using it right away and rinse with water. Consult a doctor before trying new skin remedies if you have health concerns.

Citrus-Papaya Glow Mask

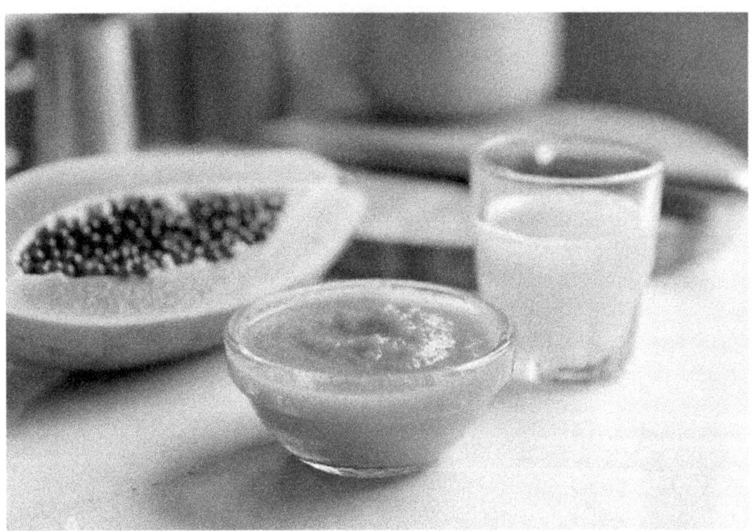

What You'll Need:

- A small chunk of ripe papaya (about a quarter of the fruit), pureed until smooth
- 1 teaspoon of fresh-squeezed lemon juice

Steps to Prepare:

1. Blend the pureed papaya together with the lemon juice in a bowl until well combined.
2. Spread the mixture evenly over your clean face, leaving it on for about 15 minutes before washing off with cool water.

Suggested Usage:

Apply this mask up to two times per week to help even out skin tone and add a natural radiance.

Important Cautions:

Skip this if your skin tends to react badly to citrus fruits, as it might cause irritation. Always do a patch test on your arm first.

Soothing Herbal Infusion for Throat Comfort

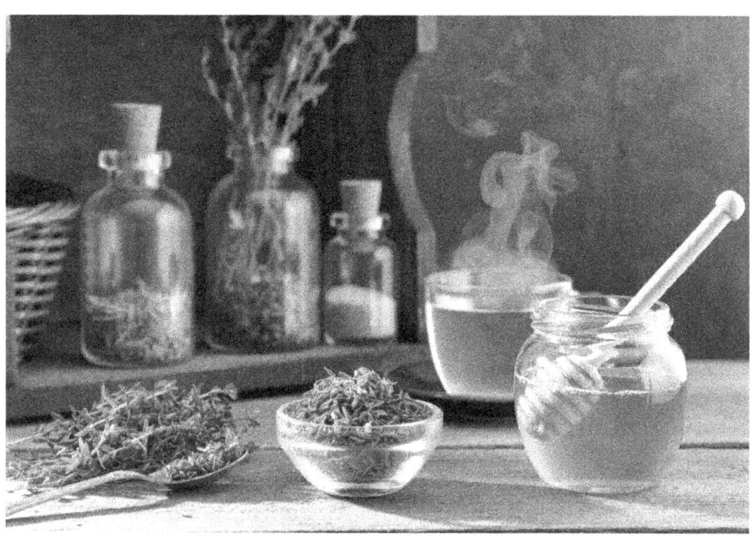

What You'll Need:

- 1 tablespoon of fresh thyme leaves
- 1 tablespoon of pure honey
- 1 cup of boiling water

Steps to Prepare:

1. Add the thyme leaves to a mug and cover them with the boiling water. Allow the mixture to rest undisturbed for around 10 minutes to draw out the natural essences.
2. Pour the liquid through a fine mesh strainer to remove the leaves, then blend in the honey until it's fully incorporated.

Suggested Usage:

Take small, warm sips throughout the day to help calm an irritated throat.

Important Cautions:

Skip this if you know you're sensitive to thyme or plants in the mint family. Always check with a healthcare provider if symptoms persist.

Green Tea Revitalizing Face Mask

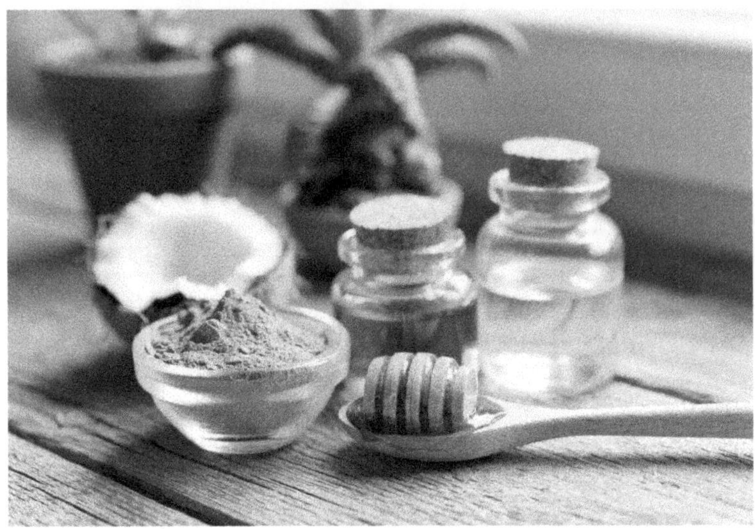

What You'll Need:

- 1 teaspoon green tea powder
- 1 tablespoon raw honey
- 1 teaspoon coconut oil

Steps to Prepare:

1. Combine the green tea powder with the raw honey in a small bowl.
2. Gently stir in the coconut oil until everything forms a creamy mixture.
3. Spread the blend evenly over your clean face, avoiding the eye area.
4. Relax and let it sit for about 15 minutes before rinsing off with warm water.

Suggested Usage:

Apply this mask once a week to help nourish your skin and promote a youthful glow.

Important Cautions:

Always do a small test on your inner arm first to check for any redness or discomfort before using it on your face.

Berry and Herb Cooling Facial Mist

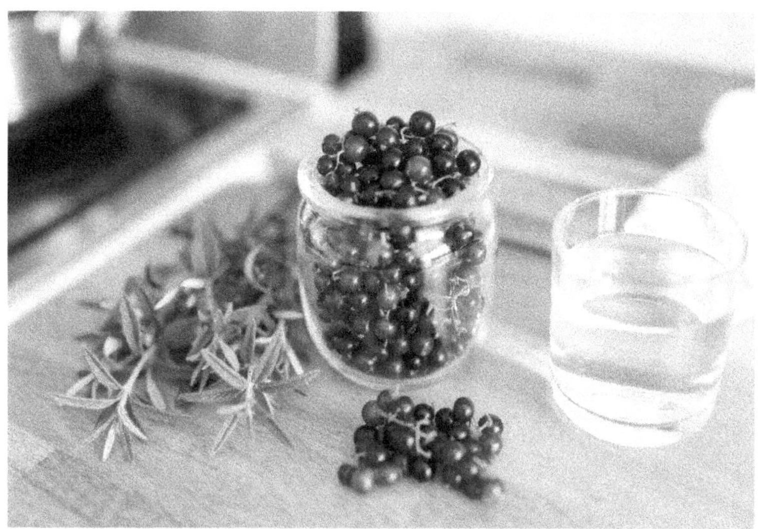

What You'll Need:

- A handful of ripe berries (about 1/2 cup)
- A small bunch of fresh herb leaves (around 1/4 cup)
- 1 cup of pure, filtered water

Steps to Prepare:

1. Gently crush the berries and herb leaves in a bowl to release their natural juices and aromas.
2. Pour in the water, stir well, and let the mixture sit for 10-15 minutes to infuse.
3. Filter the liquid through a fine mesh or clean cloth to remove any solids.
4. Transfer the clear solution into a clean spray container for easy use.

Suggested Usage:

Spray lightly over your face whenever you need a quick, invigorating pick-me-up, keeping your eyes closed.

Important Cautions:

Skip this if you have sensitivities to fruits or common garden herbs; always test a small area first.

Soothing Blend for Dry Hands

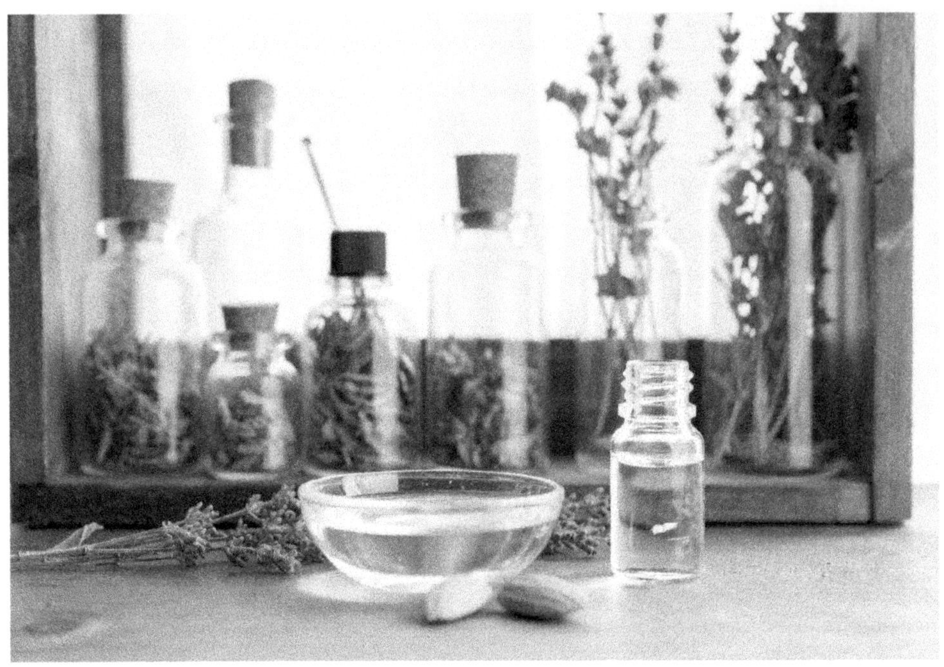

What You'll Need:

- 2 tablespoons sweet almond oil
- 5 drops lavender essential oil

Steps to Prepare:

1. Pour the sweet almond oil into a clean, small container.
2. Add the lavender essential oil and stir gently until fully combined.

Suggested Usage:

Rub a small amount onto your hands each day, working it in with light circular motions to nourish and calm the skin.

Important Cautions:

Always perform a small skin test on your inner arm first to ensure no irritation occurs.

Important Cautions:

Do not try this if you know you react badly to ginger or turmeric, as it could cause discomfort or an allergic response. Always check with a doctor if you're unsure about new foods.

Herb-Infused Scalp Soother

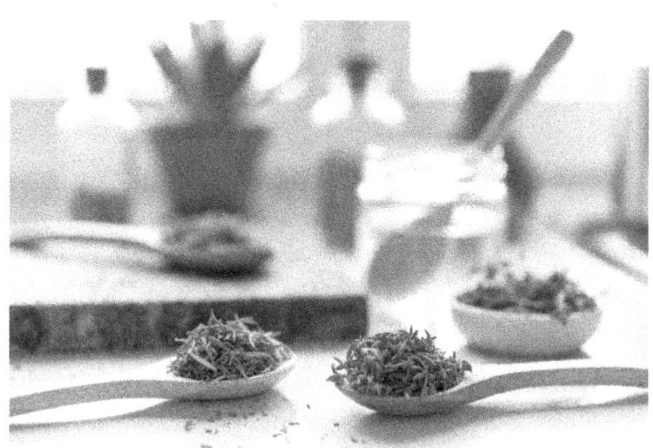

What You'll Need:

- 2 tablespoons dried rosemary leaves
- 2 tablespoons dried thyme leaves
- 1/2 cup coconut oil

Steps to Prepare:

1. Warm the coconut oil in a small pan over low heat until it melts completely.
2. Stir in the dried rosemary and thyme, letting them steep in the warm oil for about 15 minutes while keeping the heat very low.
3. Remove from heat, allow to cool slightly, then strain out the herbs using a fine mesh sieve or cheesecloth.

Suggested Usage:

Gently rub the infused oil into your scalp using your fingertips in circular motions for around 5-7 minutes. Let it sit for 20-40 minutes to absorb, then rinse thoroughly with your regular shampoo.

Important Cautions:

Do a small skin test first to check for any irritation. Skip this if you're expecting a baby or have known reactions to strong herbal scents or oils.

Citrus Spice Foot Polish

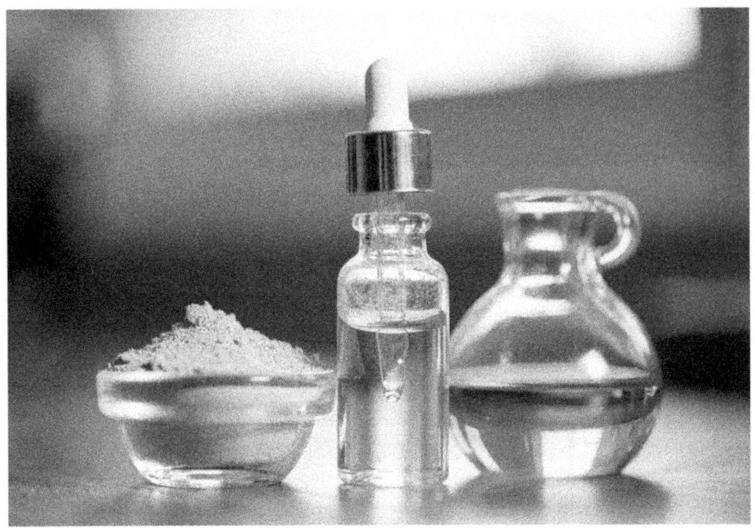

What You'll Need:

- 1 tablespoon finely powdered cloves
- 1 tablespoon fresh-squeezed citrus extract (from a lemon)
- 1 tablespoon natural plant oil (like from olives)

Steps to Prepare:

1. Combine the powdered cloves with the citrus extract and plant oil in a small dish.
2. Stir everything together until it forms a smooth, spreadable paste.

Suggested Usage:

Apply the mixture to your feet with light circular motions to remove rough patches, then rinse off with warm water. Try this routine every seven days for smoother skin.

Important Cautions:

Always do a small patch test on your skin first to check for any sensitivity or redness.

Nourishing Autumn Squash Face Blend

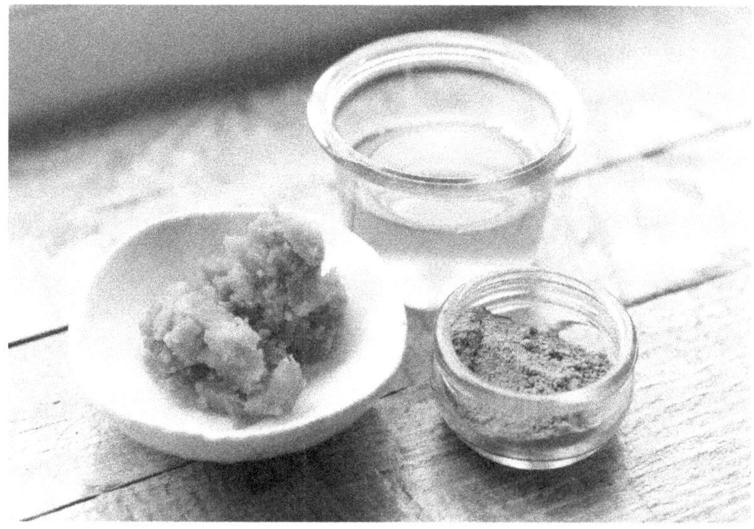

What You'll Need:

- 3 tablespoons of fresh mashed squash (from a cooked pumpkin)
- Half a teaspoon of ground spice bark (cinnamon)
- 2 teaspoons of raw bee nectar (honey)

Steps to Prepare:

1. Stir the mashed squash, ground spice, and bee nectar together in a small bowl until you get a creamy mixture.
2. Spread an even layer over your clean face, avoiding the eyes, and let it sit for about 15 minutes.
3. Rinse off gently with warm water and pat dry.

Suggested Usage:

Apply this blend once or twice each week to help refresh and brighten your complexion naturally.

Important Cautions:

Always try a small test spot on your arm first to make sure it doesn't cause any redness or discomfort, especially if you have sensitive skin.

Refreshing Morning Cleanse Beverage

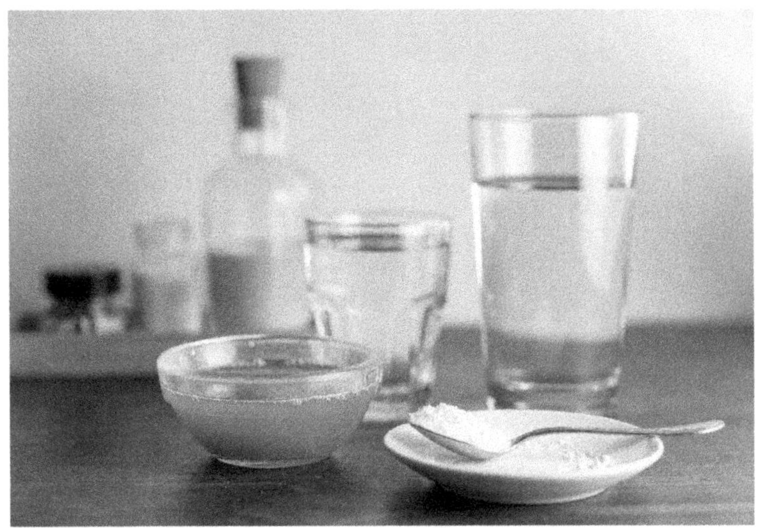

What You'll Need:

- 1 tablespoon of raw apple cider vinegar
- 1/4 teaspoon of sodium bicarbonate (commonly known as baking soda)
- 8 ounces of room-temperature filtered water

Steps to Prepare:

1. Pour the water into a clean glass.
2. Add the apple cider vinegar followed by the sodium bicarbonate.
3. Mix thoroughly until the fizzing subsides, then sip slowly.

Suggested Usage:

Consume this first thing upon waking to support your body's natural cleansing processes.

Important Cautions:

Skip this if you experience heartburn or stomach acid issues, and consult a healthcare provider before starting any new routine.

Soothing Spice Infusion for Tummy Relief

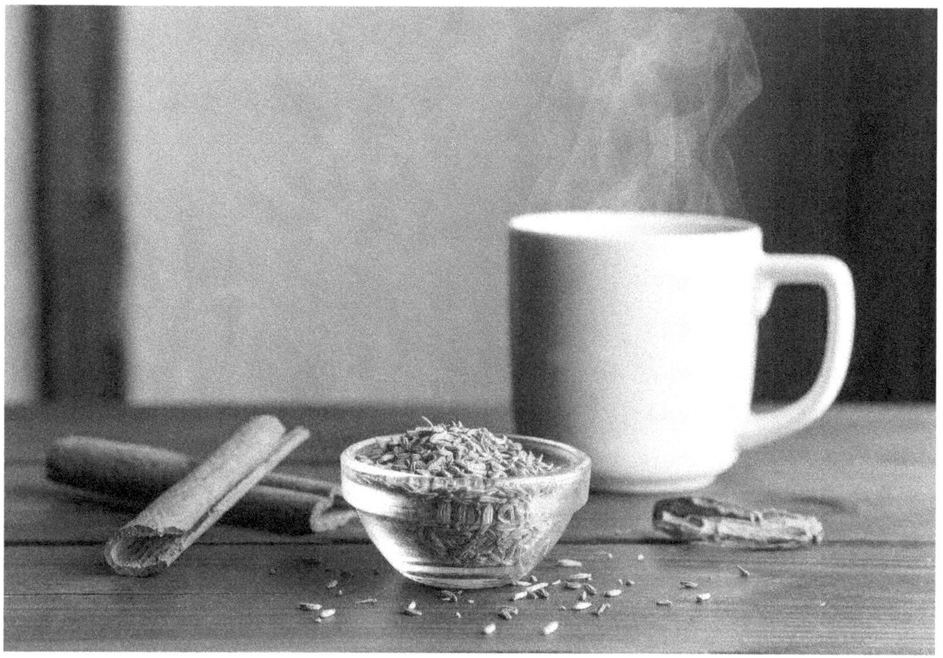

What You'll Need:

- 1 teaspoon crushed fennel seeds
- 1 small piece of cinnamon bark
- 1 mug of fresh hot water

Steps to Prepare:

1. Place the crushed seeds and bark piece into a small saucepan with the water.
2. Heat on low until it simmers gently for about 5 minutes.
3. Pour through a sieve into your mug, then take small sips while it's warm.

Suggested Usage:

Enjoy a cup right after eating to help settle your stomach.

Important Cautions:

Skip this if you react badly to fennel or similar spices.

Soothing Aromatic Balm for Breathing Ease

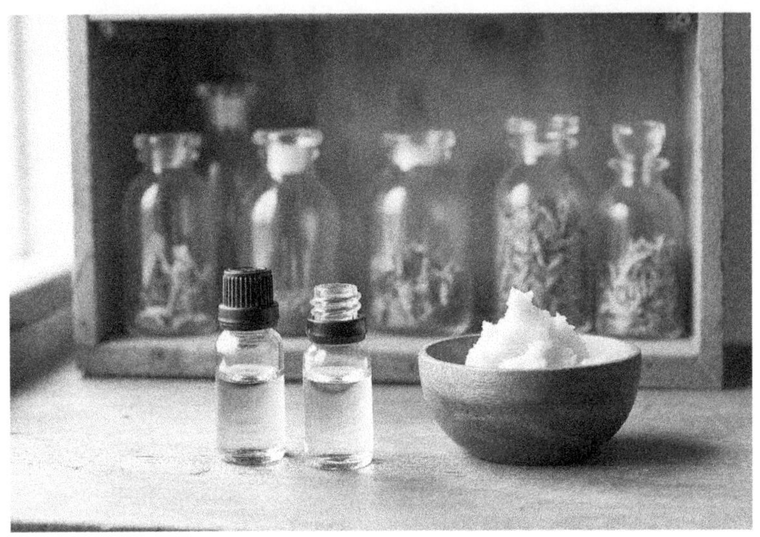

What You'll Need:

- 1 tablespoon of lavender essential oil
- 1 tablespoon of eucalyptus essential oil
- 1 tablespoon of melted shea butter (as a gentle base)

Steps to Prepare:

1. Gently warm the shea butter until it's soft and liquid.
2. Stir in the lavender and eucalyptus oils until fully blended.
3. Let the mixture cool slightly before storing in a small jar.

Suggested Usage:

Rub a small amount onto your upper chest area each evening to help clear stuffy airways and promote restful sleep.

Important Cautions:

Do not apply this to babies or toddlers, and skip it if you're expecting a child, as strong scents might cause irritation.

Soothing Root and Spice Beverage for Easing Body Discomfort

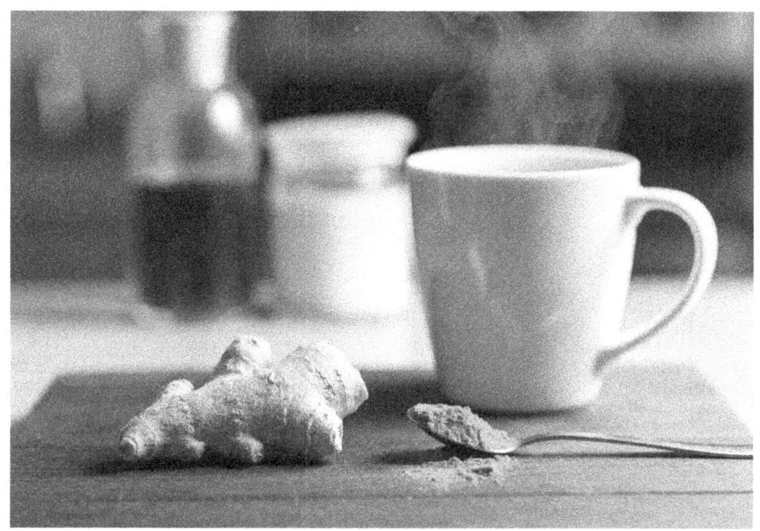

What You'll Need:

- A small piece of raw ginger (about the size of your thumb)
- A pinch of powdered golden spice (around half a small spoon)
- A spoonful of natural sweetener like bee nectar
- A mugful of comfortably hot liquid

Steps to Prepare:

1. Peel and finely shred the ginger piece, then blend it with the golden spice and sweetener until it forms a smooth paste.
2. Pour the hot liquid over the mixture and whisk briskly to combine everything evenly.

Suggested Usage:

Sip this warm drink once each day to help calm everyday aches and promote a sense of ease in your system.

Important Cautions:

Skip this if you have a known sensitivity to the root or spice components, and check with a health expert if you're expecting, nursing, or on medications.

Cooling Cucumber Aloe Soother

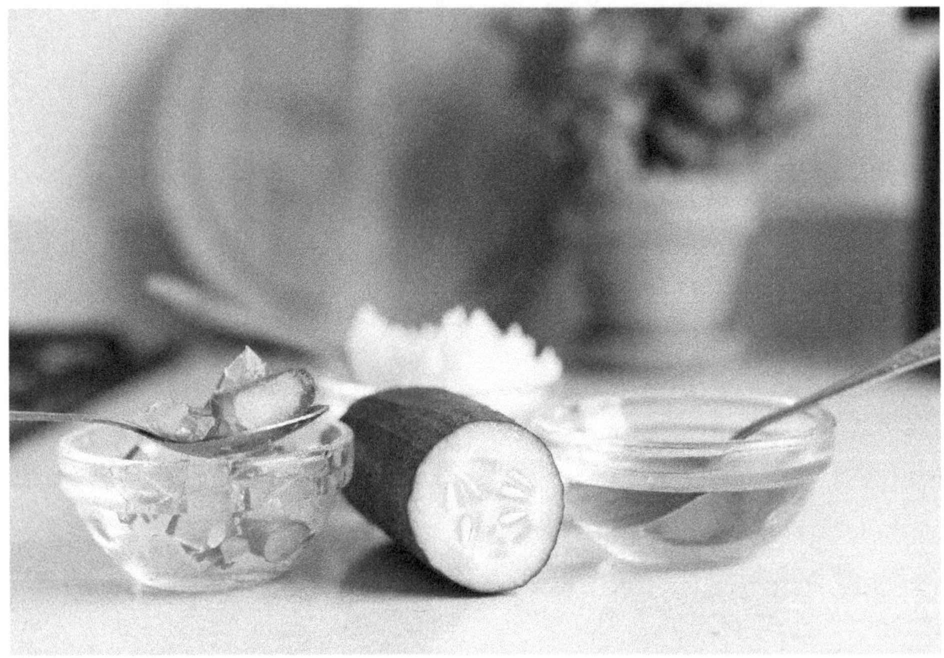

What You'll Need:

- Half a fresh cucumber, pureed
- Two spoonfuls of pure aloe vera gel
- One small spoonful of natural vitamin E oil

Steps to Prepare:

1. Puree the cucumber until it's smooth and juicy.
2. Combine the puree with the aloe vera gel and stir in the vitamin E oil until everything blends evenly.
3. Spread the mixture gently on your skin to refresh and moisturize.

Suggested Usage:

Let it sit on your face for about 15 to 20 minutes, then wash off with cool water.

Important Cautions:

Always try a small dab on your inner arm first to check for any irritation.

Soothing Oats and Nectar Bath Blend

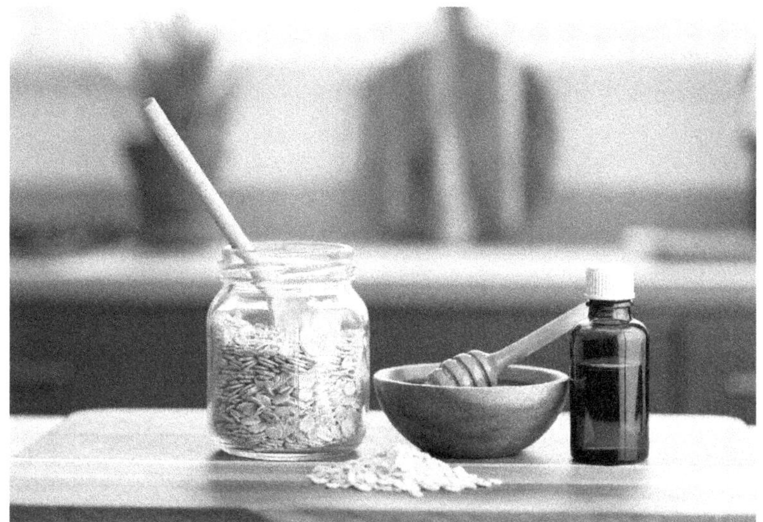

What You'll Need:

- 3/4 cup rolled oats
- 1 tablespoon raw honey
- 4 drops chamomile essential oil

Steps to Prepare:

1. Pulse the rolled oats in a blender until they form a soft dust.
2. Warm the honey slightly to make it easier to stir, then combine it with the oat dust and chamomile oil in a bowl.
3. Stir everything together until well blended, then pour the mixture directly into running bath water.

Suggested Usage:

Relax in the tub for about 15 minutes to calm irritated skin and promote a sense of peace.

Important Cautions:

Test for sensitivity to chamomile by applying a small amount to your inner arm first; stop use if any redness or discomfort occurs.

Herbal Boost Syrup with Coneflower and Berries

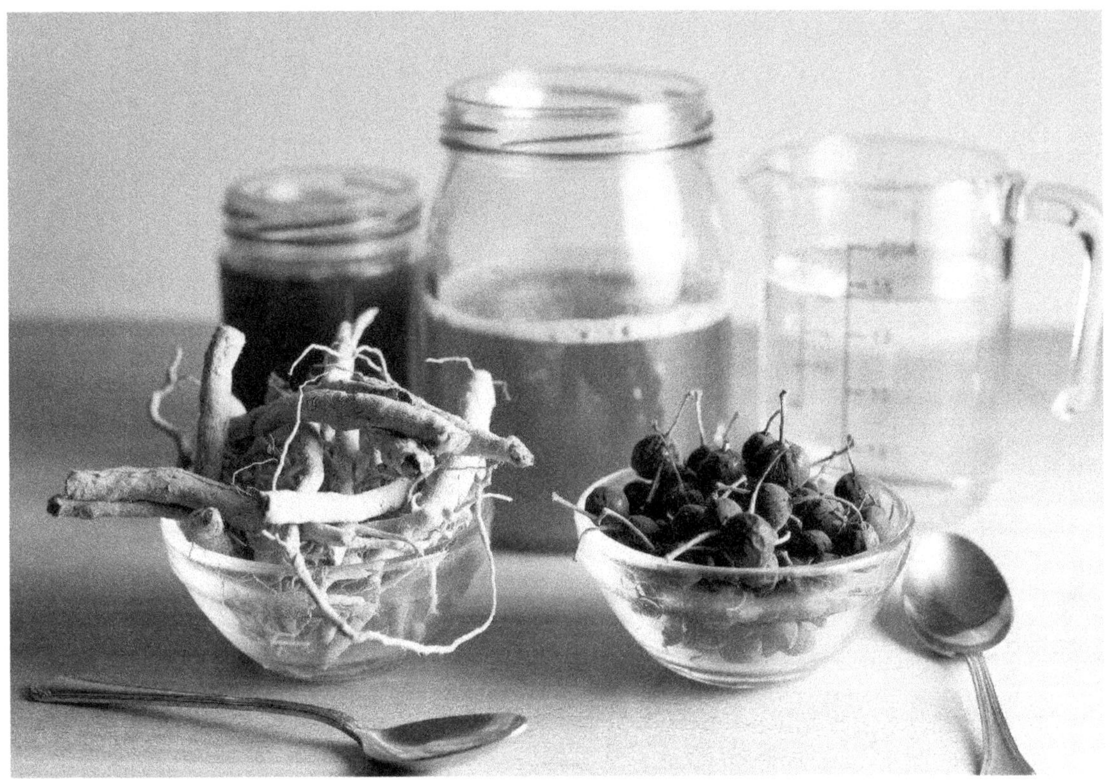

What You'll Need:

- 2 teaspoons of dried coneflower roots
- 2 teaspoons of dried elder fruits
- 8 ounces of pure honey
- 8 ounces of clean water

Steps to Prepare:

1. Pour the water into a small pot and add the coneflower roots and elder fruits.
2. Heat the mixture on a low flame until it starts to simmer gently, then let it continue for about 20 minutes to draw out the natural essences.
3. Remove from the stove, allow it to cool slightly, then pour through a fine mesh to separate the liquid from the plant parts.
4. Stir in the honey until it blends smoothly with the warm herbal liquid.
5. Transfer to a clean jar and store in a cool spot.

Suggested Usage:

Consume one teaspoon each morning to help support your body's natural defenses against everyday challenges.

Important Cautions:

Skip this if you're expecting or nursing a baby, as it might not be suitable during those times. Always check with a health expert if you have any concerns.

Calming Herb Pouch for Restful Nights

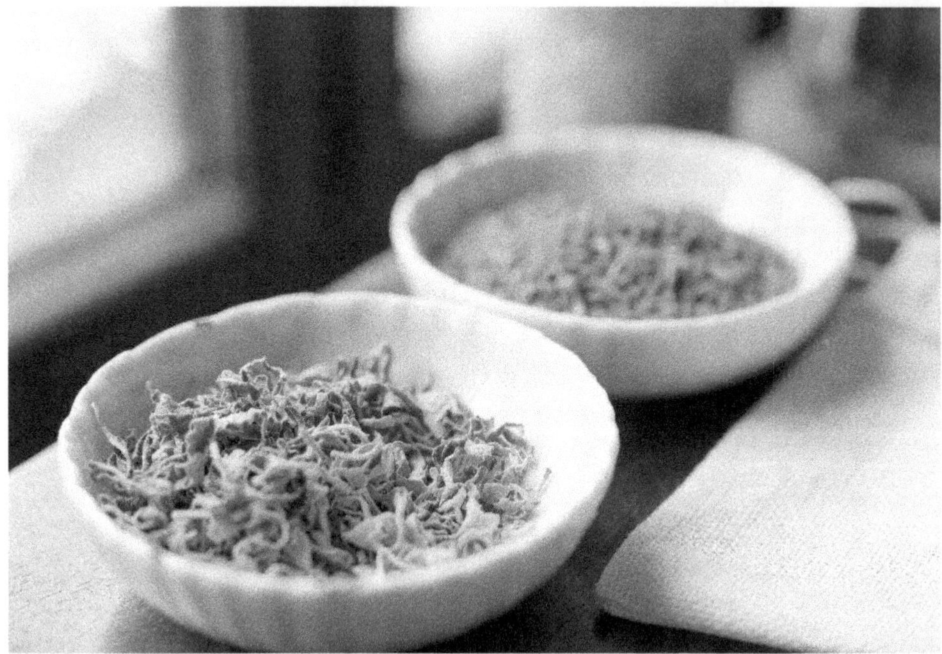

What You'll Need:

- 2 tablespoons of dried lemon balm leaves
- 2 tablespoons of dried lavender buds
- A small muslin bag or fabric pouch

Steps to Prepare:

1. Gently blend the lemon balm leaves and lavender buds in a clean bowl.
2. Spoon the herb mixture into the muslin bag, then secure it tightly with a drawstring or knot.

Suggested Usage:

Tuck the pouch inside your pillowcase or set it on your nightstand to help promote a calm and soothing atmosphere for sleep.

Important Cautions:

Consult a healthcare provider before use if you are pregnant, as some herbs may affect you differently during this time.

Soothing Blossom Infused Oil for Skin Repair

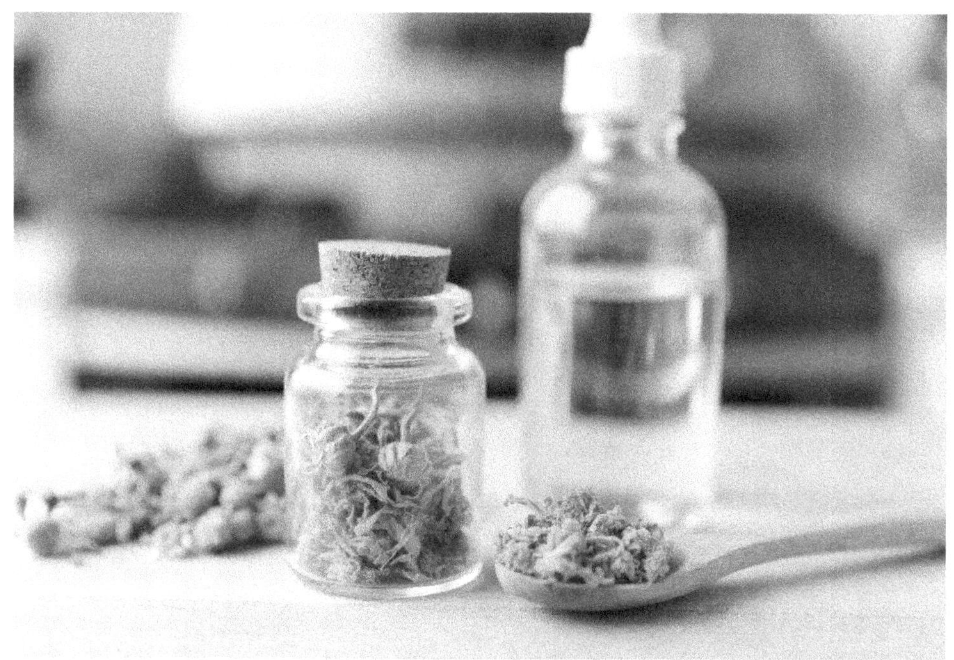

What You'll Need:

- 2 tablespoons dried marigold blossoms (calendula)
- 1 tablespoon dried chamomile blooms
- 1/3 cup carrier oil, such as jojoba or almond oil

Steps to Prepare:

1. Combine the dried blossoms and blooms in a clean glass jar.
2. Pour the carrier oil over the plant materials until fully covered.
3. Seal the jar tightly and place it in a warm, sunny spot for about 10 days, shaking gently each day to mix.
4. After the time is up, filter out the solids using a fine mesh strainer or cheesecloth.
5. Transfer the clear oil to an amber glass container for storage, keeping it away from direct light.

Suggested Usage:

Gently massage a small amount onto clean, affected skin areas to support natural recovery and comfort.

Important Cautions:

Always do a small skin test on your inner arm before full use to check for any sensitivity. Stop using if irritation occurs, and consult a doctor if you have known plant allergies or ongoing skin issues.

Garlic and Cayenne Warm Drink for Enhanced Blood Flow

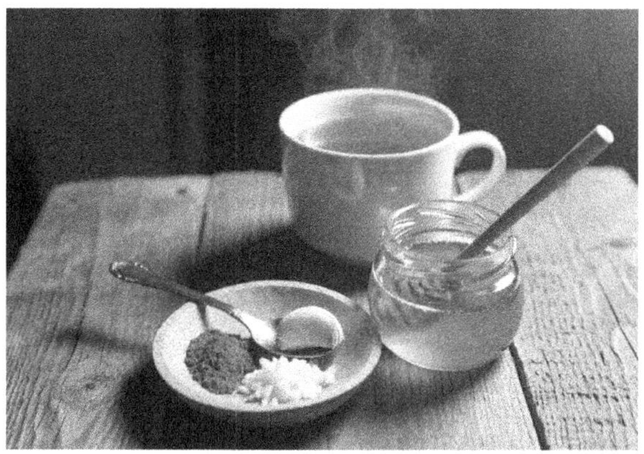

What You'll Need:

- A small dash (about 1/4 teaspoon) of cayenne powder
- One fresh garlic clove, finely chopped
- A spoonful (around 1 tablespoon) of raw honey
- 1 full cup of heated water

Steps to Prepare:

1. Chop the garlic into small pieces and let it rest for a few minutes to activate its natural benefits.
2. Add the cayenne powder and honey to a mug.
3. Pour in the heated water and stir everything together until fully blended.

Suggested Usage:

Sip one mug each day, preferably in the morning, to support smoother blood movement throughout your body.

Important Cautions:

Steer clear if you react badly to hot spices or have stomach troubles like ulcers. Always talk to a healthcare provider before starting, especially if you're on medications or have health conditions.

Calming Blend Tea for Tension Relief

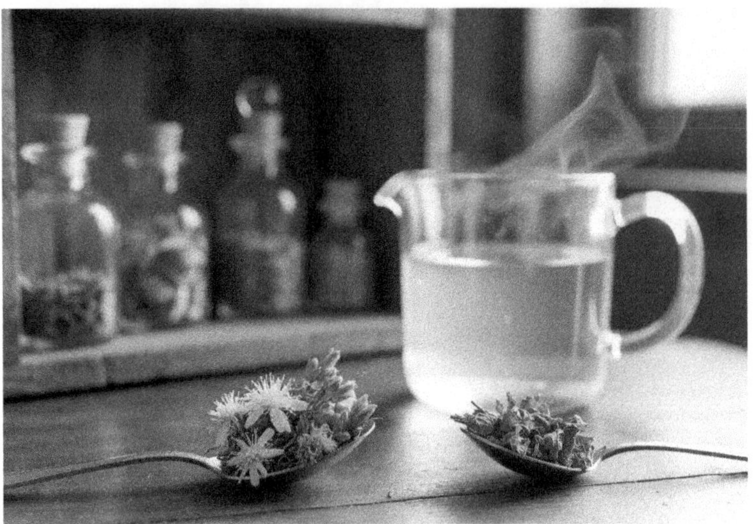

What You'll Need:

- A teaspoon of dried St. John's wort blossoms
- A teaspoon of dried mint foliage
- Eight ounces of freshly heated water

Steps to Prepare:

1. Combine the dried blossoms and foliage in a cup or infuser.
2. Add the hot water, ensuring it's not still bubbling to preserve the gentle flavors.
3. Cover and allow the mixture to infuse for around eight to twelve minutes.
4. Remove the plant material with a strainer.
5. Take small sips while it's still warm.

Suggested Usage:

Enjoy a single serving during moments of unease to help foster a sense of ease and calm.

Important Cautions:

Speak with a medical professional prior to trying this if you use any prescribed drugs, since St. John's wort might affect how they work in your body.

Citrus Ginger Cleansing Blend

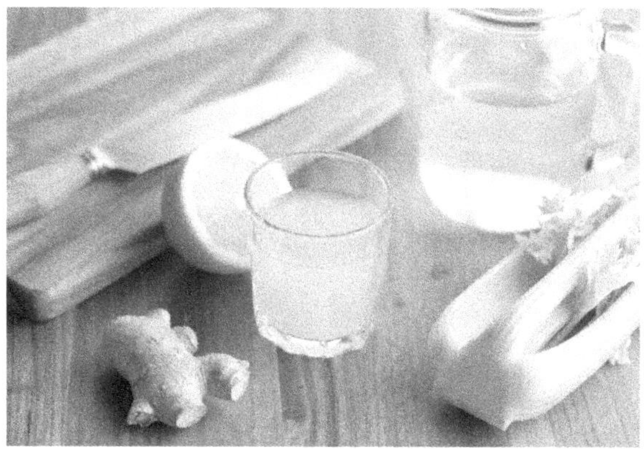

What You'll Need:

- Fresh juice from one medium lemon
- A thumb-sized piece of fresh ginger
- Half a medium celery stalk
- 1 cup of filtered water

Steps to Prepare:

1. Peel the ginger and chop it into small chunks.
2. Cut the celery into pieces.
3. Combine the lemon juice, ginger chunks, celery pieces, and water in a blender.
4. Mix on high speed until everything is fully combined and silky.
5. Pour into a glass right away.

Suggested Usage:

Sip this refreshing drink first thing each day to help flush out toxins and kickstart your system.

Important Cautions:

Skip this if you're sensitive to citrus fruits, and check with a doctor if you have stomach issues or are on medications.

Azadirachta Leaf and Golden Spice Blemish Blend

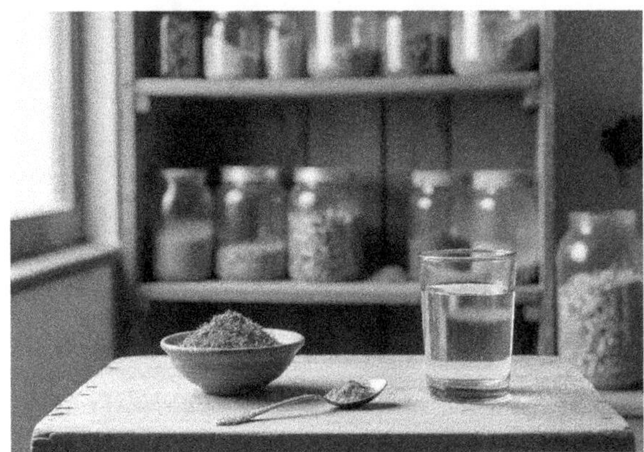

What You'll Need:

- 2 teaspoons of ground azadirachta (neem) leaves
- 1/4 teaspoon of golden spice (turmeric) powder
- A splash of clean water (about 1-2 teaspoons, as needed)

Steps to Prepare:

1. Start by combining the ground azadirachta leaves and golden spice in a small dish.
2. Gradually stir in the water until you form a smooth, spreadable mixture that's not too runny.

Suggested Usage:

Dab the blend onto problem spots on your skin and let it sit for 10-20 minutes, then gently wash off with lukewarm water. Try this once a day for clearer-looking skin over time.

Important Cautions:

Test a small area first to check for irritation, especially if you have sensitive skin or known reactions to spices like turmeric. Avoid getting it in your eyes, and consult a doctor if blemishes worsen.

Soothing Chest Rub for Clearer Breathing

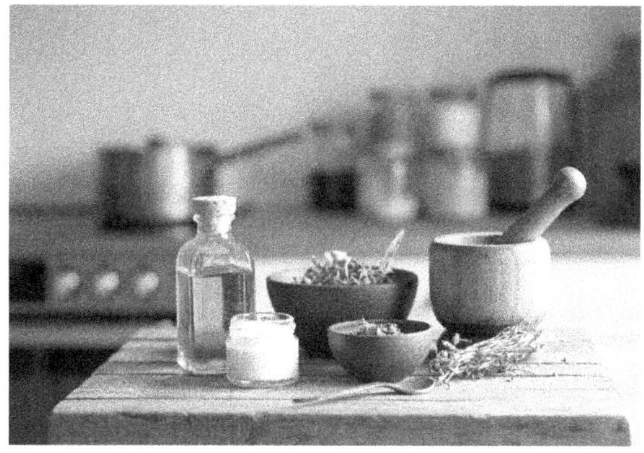

What You'll Need:

- 1 tablespoon eucalyptus essential oil
- 1 tablespoon peppermint essential oil
- 1/4 cup shea butter
- 1 teaspoon beeswax pellets (optional, for a firmer texture)

Steps to Prepare:

1. Gently heat the shea butter and beeswax (if using) in a small pot over low heat until fully liquid.
2. Remove from heat and stir in the eucalyptus and peppermint essential oils until well blended.
3. Pour the mixture into a clean container and let it cool completely to set.

Suggested Usage:

Gently massage a small amount onto your upper chest area to help ease breathing discomfort.

Important Cautions:

Keep away from sensitive areas like the eyes and mouth. Always do a patch test on your skin first to check for any irritation. Consult a doctor if you have breathing issues or are pregnant.

Nigella and Lavender Calming Face Blend

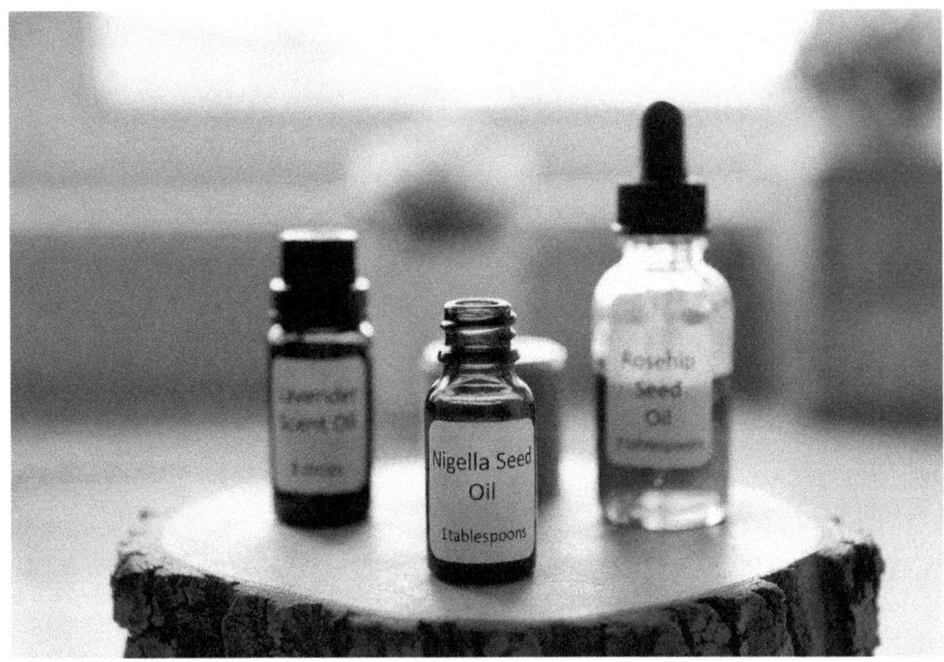

What You'll Need:

- 1 tablespoon nigella seed oil (also known as black cumin seed oil)
- 3 drops lavender scent oil
- 2 tablespoons rosehip seed oil

Steps to Prepare:

1. Pour the nigella seed oil and rosehip seed oil into a clean glass container.
2. Add the lavender scent oil and gently swirl to combine everything evenly.
3. Seal the container tightly.

Suggested Usage:

Gently massage 2-3 drops onto your clean face each evening before sleep.

Important Cautions:

Always try a small dab on your inner arm first to make sure your skin doesn't react badly. Avoid it if you're pregnant or have known allergies to these plants.

Energizing Root and Nectar Infusion

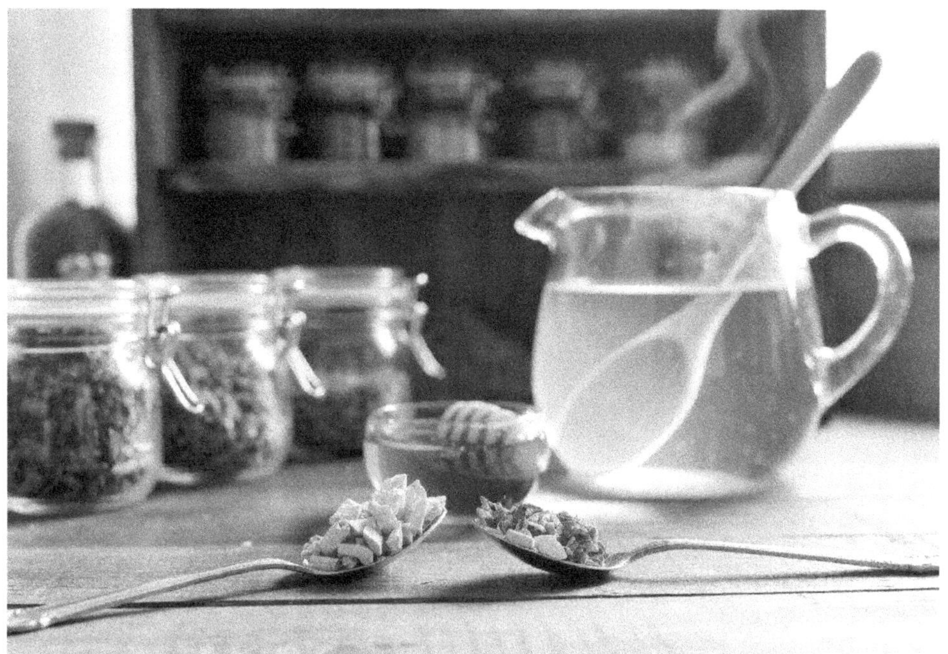

What You'll Need:

- 2 teaspoons chopped dry ginseng pieces
- 2 teaspoons natural sweetener like honey
- 8 ounces boiling water

Steps to Prepare:

1. Place the ginseng pieces in a mug and pour the boiling water over them.
2. Let it sit covered for about 8-12 minutes to draw out the flavors.
3. Mix in the sweetener until it dissolves completely, then sip slowly.

Suggested Usage:

Enjoy a cup first thing after waking to help sharpen focus and alertness throughout the day.

Important Cautions:

Skip this if you're expecting a baby or taking specific drugs, and check with a healthcare provider first.

Refreshing Citrus Herb Infusion

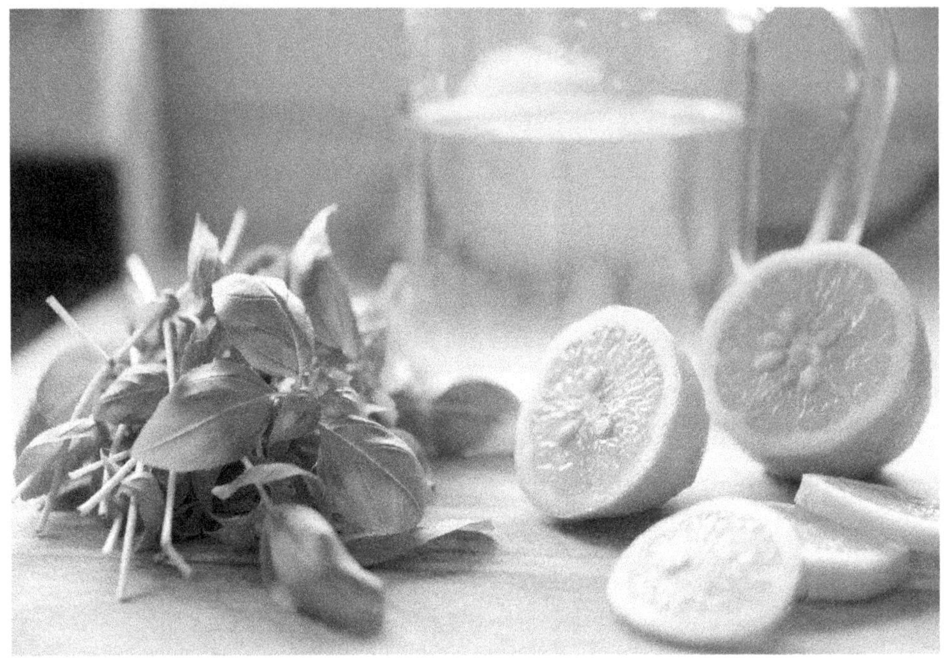

What You'll Need:

- A handful of fresh basil sprigs
- One whole lemon, cut into thin rounds
- About 4 cups of clean, filtered water

Steps to Prepare:

1. Gently rinse the basil and lemon under cool water to remove any dirt.
2. Place the basil sprigs and lemon rounds into a large pitcher or jar.
3. Pour in the water, then cover and let it sit in the refrigerator overnight to allow the flavors to blend.

Suggested Usage:

Sip on this throughout your daily routine to help support your body's natural cleansing processes and stay hydrated.

Important Cautions:

Always confirm you have no sensitivities to citrus fruits or herbs like basil before trying this. If you notice any unusual reactions, stop using it right away.

Tropical Nutty Fruit Drink for Skin Vitality

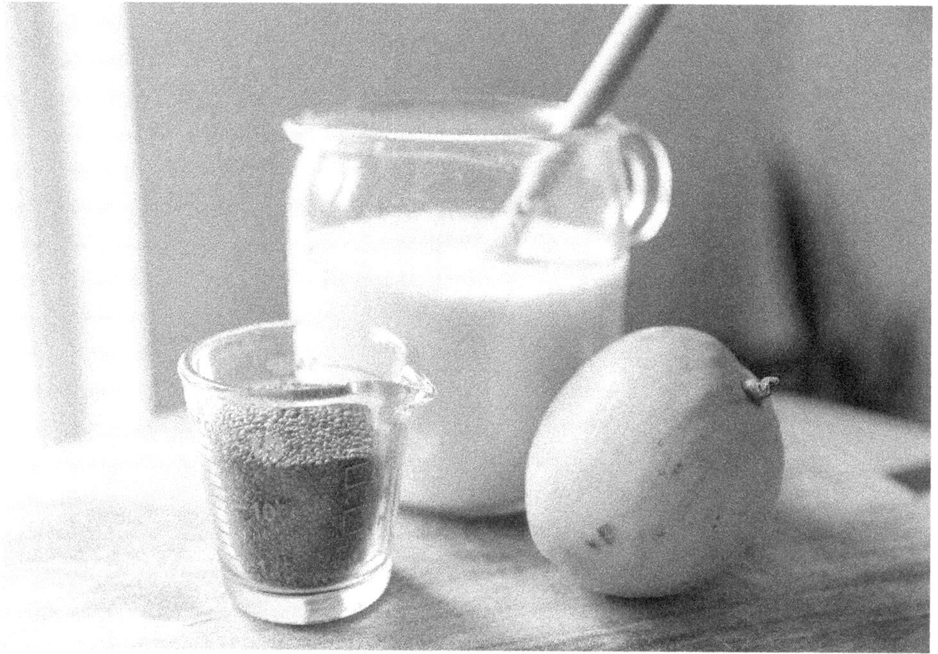

What You'll Need:

- 1/3 cup small black seeds (like chia)
- 1 medium soft tropical fruit (such as mango)
- 3/4 cup plant-based liquid (for example, from coconuts)

Steps to Prepare:

1. Let the seeds sit in a bit of water for about 10 minutes to soften them up.
2. Peel and chop the fruit into small pieces.
3. Mix the softened seeds, fruit chunks, and liquid in a mixer until it's all creamy and even.

Suggested Usage:

Enjoy this drink once or twice every seven days as part of your routine.

Important Cautions:

Always soften the seeds in liquid first to make them easier on your stomach and avoid any discomfort. If you have allergies to fruits or nuts, check with a doctor before trying.

Soothing Ginger-Fennel Drink for Better Digestion

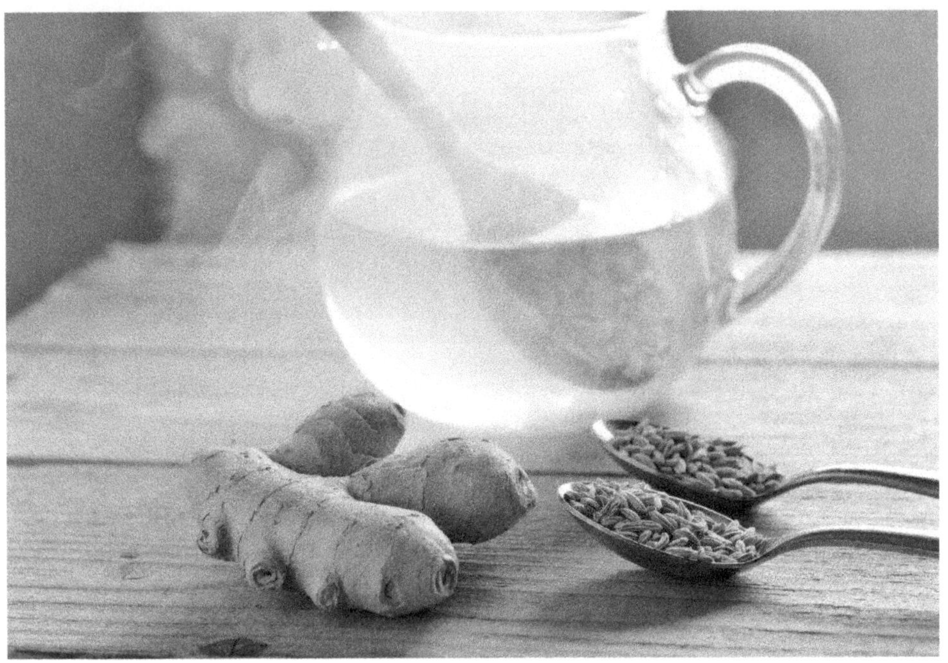

What You'll Need:

- A thumb-sized piece of fresh ginger
- 2 teaspoons fennel seeds
- 8 ounces boiling water

Steps to Prepare:

1. Rinse the ginger and cut it into thin slices.
2. Gently crush the fennel seeds using a spoon or mortar to help release their natural flavors.
3. Add the sliced ginger and crushed seeds to a heat-safe cup.
4. Pour the boiling water over them and cover the cup to keep the heat in.
5. Allow the mixture to brew for about 8 to 12 minutes.
6. Pour through a fine mesh strainer to remove the pieces, then let it cool slightly before drinking.

Suggested Usage:

Enjoy one cup right after eating to help calm your stomach and support easy food processing.

Important Cautions:

Stay away from this if you're sensitive to fennel or similar herbs like dill or carrot. Talk to a doctor first if you're expecting a baby, nursing, or dealing with any stomach problems.

Stinging Nettle and Dandelion Cleansing Infusion

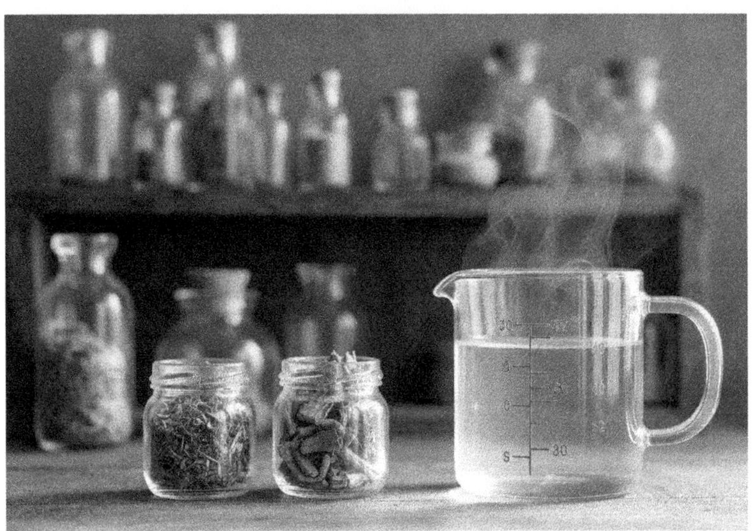

What You'll Need:

- 2 teaspoons of dried stinging nettle leaves
- 1 teaspoon of dried dandelion root pieces
- 8 ounces of freshly boiled water

Steps to Prepare:

1. Add the nettle leaves and dandelion root to a mug or teapot.
2. Pour the boiled water over the mixture.
3. Cover and allow it to infuse for about 15 minutes.
4. Use a fine mesh strainer to remove the plant material before sipping.

Suggested Usage:

Enjoy one cup each morning to help your body flush out toxins and support overall kidney function.

Important Cautions:

Speak with a healthcare professional before trying this if you're using medications that thin the blood, as it might interact.

Spicy Defense Elixir

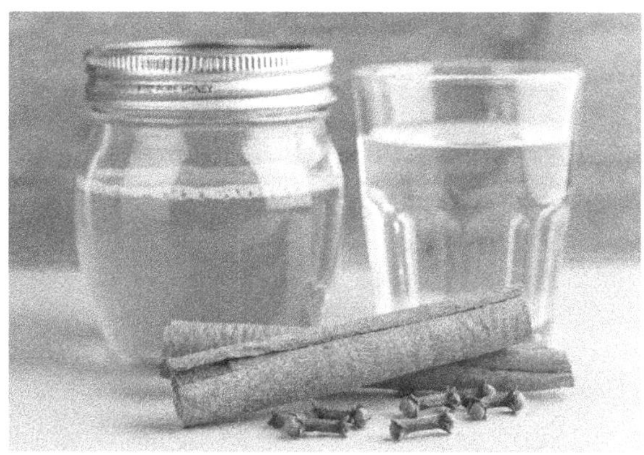

What You'll Need:

- A single cinnamon bark piece
- Six whole clove buds
- Eight ounces of pure honey
- Four ounces of clean water

Steps to Prepare:

1. Pour the water into a small pot, add the cinnamon bark and clove buds, and heat until it reaches a soft boil.
2. Lower the flame and allow the mix to gently simmer for about 12 minutes to release the warming essences.
3. Take it off the stove, pour through a fine mesh to remove the solids, and stir in the honey until it fully blends and cools down.

Suggested Usage:

Stir one tablespoon into warm tea or take it straight each morning to help fortify your body's natural protections.

Important Cautions:

Skip this for babies under 12 months old, since raw honey might carry health risks for them. Always check with a doctor if you have spice sensitivities or are expecting.

Soothing Arnica Lavender Balm for Muscle Discomfort

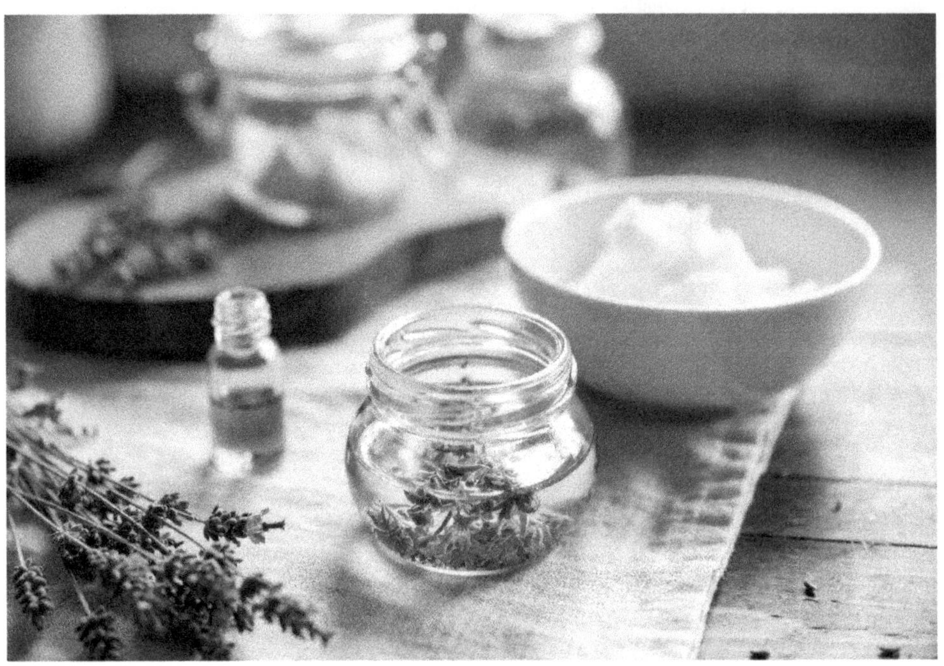

What You'll Need:

- 2 tablespoons of oil infused with arnica flowers
- A couple of drops of pure lavender oil from the plant
- 1 tablespoon of solid coconut fat

Steps to Prepare:

1. Combine all the items in a small container until well blended.
2. Gently massage the mixture onto areas feeling tense or achy.

Suggested Usage:

Dab on whenever discomfort arises to help ease the feeling.

Important Cautions:

Steer clear of applying to any cuts or open areas on the skin.

Refreshing Mint and Citrus Mist

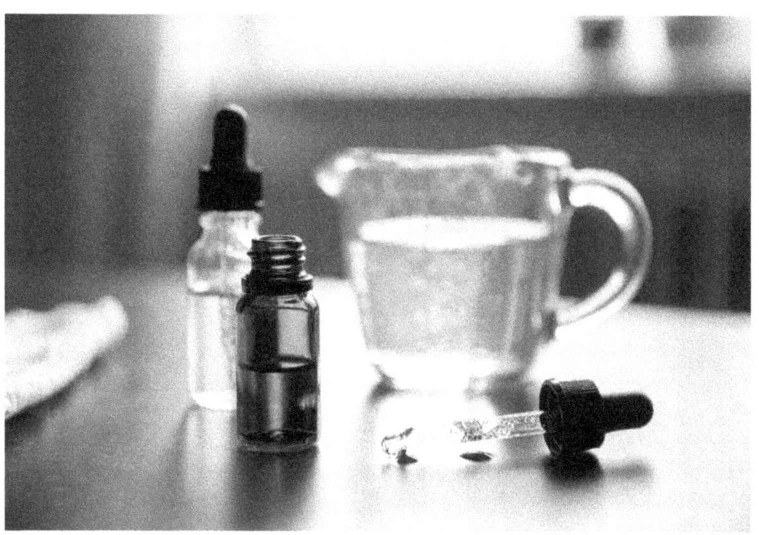

What You'll Need:

- 4 drops peppermint essential oil
- 6 drops lemon essential oil
- 1/2 cup distilled water

Steps to Prepare:

1. Pour the distilled water into a clean spray bottle.
2. Drop in the peppermint and lemon oils.
3. Close the bottle tightly and give it a good shake to blend everything together.

Suggested Usage:

Lightly mist the mixture onto your arms, legs, or neck whenever you need a quick, invigorating cool-down, like after exercise or on warm afternoons.

Important Cautions:

Steer clear of spraying near your face or sensitive areas to prevent any accidental eye irritation. Test a small patch of skin first to check for sensitivity, and stop using if redness appears.

Berry Boost and Sweet Root Defense Mixture

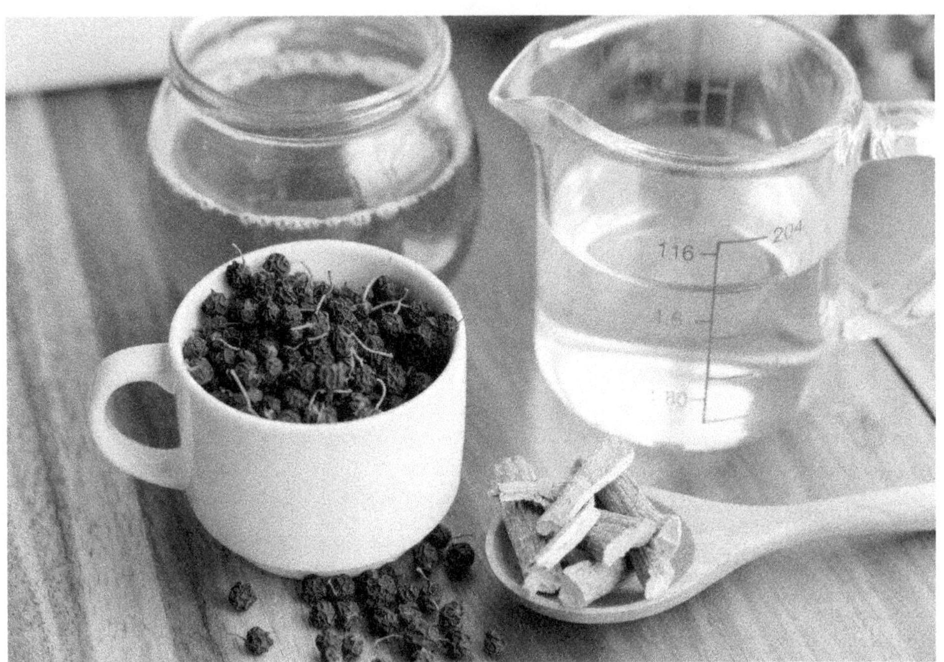

What You'll Need:

- Half a cup of dried elderberries
- One tablespoon of dried licorice root pieces
- Half a cup of raw honey
- One cup of fresh water

Steps to Prepare:

1. In a small pot, combine the elderberries, licorice root, and water, then bring to a gentle simmer over medium heat.
2. Let it cook slowly for about 25 minutes to draw out the natural essences.
3. Remove from heat, filter out the solids using a fine mesh strainer, and stir in the honey until fully blended.
4. Pour into a clean glass container and keep it in the fridge for up to two weeks.

Suggested Usage:

Consume one spoonful each day to help support your body's natural defenses.

Important Cautions:

Skip this if you have issues with elevated blood pressure, as licorice root might affect it. Always check with a doctor before starting any new herbal routine, especially if pregnant or on medications.

Golden Spice Soothing Blend

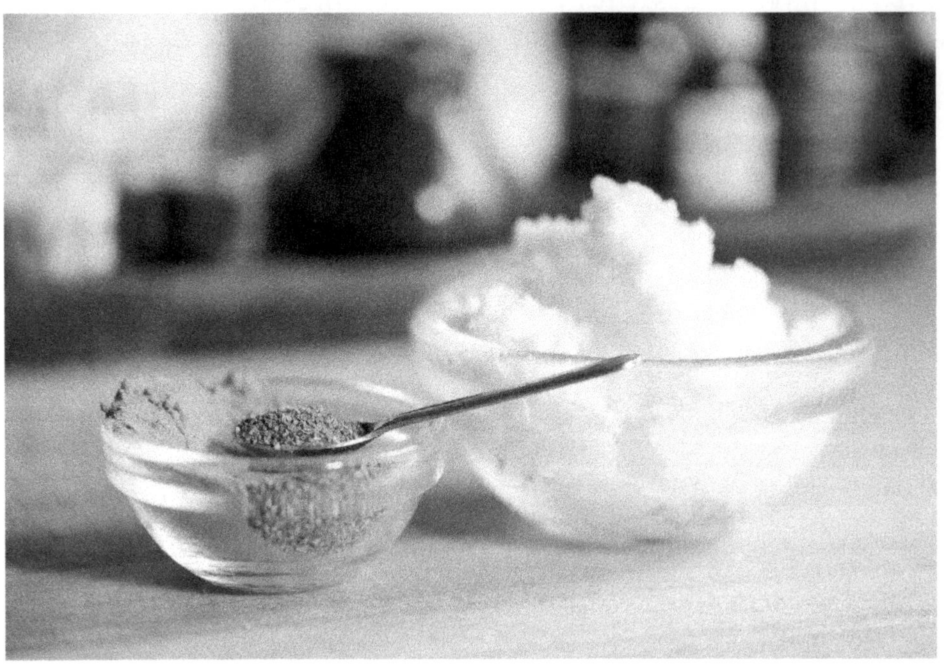

What You'll Need:

- One small spoonful of ground turmeric
- Half a small spoonful of ground black pepper
- A generous dollop of coconut oil (about one large spoonful)

Steps to Prepare:

1. Combine the turmeric and black pepper in a small bowl.
2. Stir in the coconut oil until everything forms a smooth, spreadable mixture.

Suggested Usage:

Gently rub the blend onto sore spots on your skin to help ease discomfort.

Important Cautions:

Do not apply to cuts or broken skin, as it might cause irritation. Always test a small area first to check for any sensitivity.

Calming Herb Blend Drink for Everyday Tension

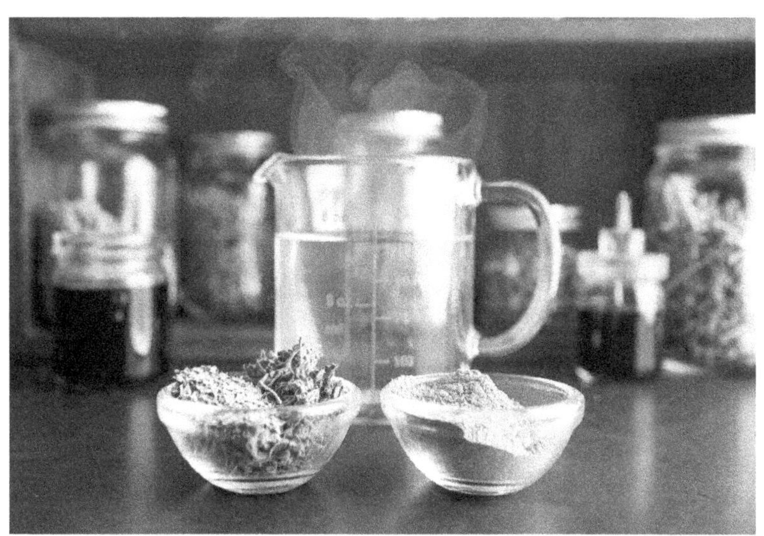

What You'll Need:

- 2 teaspoons of dried lemon balm leaves
- 1/2 teaspoon of ashwagandha root extract in powder form
- 8 ounces of fresh boiling water

Steps to Prepare:

1. Pour the boiling water over the lemon balm leaves in a mug and let it sit covered for about 7 minutes to draw out the flavors.
2. Mix in the ashwagandha powder until it fully dissolves, giving it a good stir to combine everything smoothly.

Suggested Usage:

Sip on one serving each day to help ease feelings of daily pressure and promote a sense of relaxation.

Important Cautions:

Talk to your healthcare provider first if you're expecting a baby or have any ongoing health conditions.

Soothing Spice Foot Bath

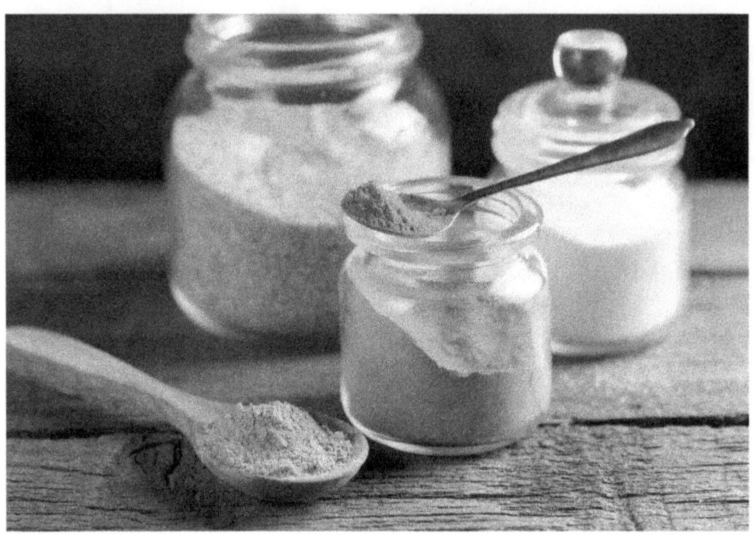

What You'll Need:

- 1 tablespoon ginger powder
- 1 tablespoon turmeric spice
- 2 cups Epsom salt
- 1/2 cup baking soda

Steps to Prepare:

1. Stir together the ginger powder, turmeric spice, Epsom salt, and baking soda in a large bowl.
2. Pour the mixture into a basin filled with comfortably warm water and blend well until dissolved.
3. Place your feet in the basin and relax for around 20 minutes.

Suggested Usage:

Enjoy this foot bath about once each week to help unwind and reduce minor swelling.

Important Cautions:

Always test the water temperature with your hand first to prevent discomfort from heat.

Nourishing Seed Gel Mask for Dry Skin

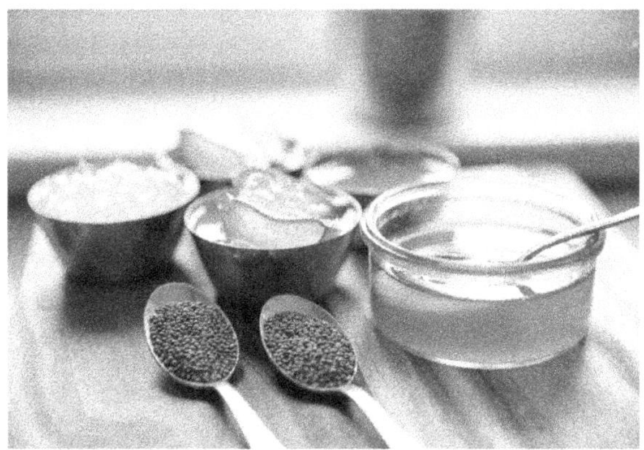

What You'll Need:

- 2 teaspoons of small black seeds (like chia)
- 3 tablespoons of clear plant gel from aloe leaves
- Half a teaspoon of natural sweet syrup (such as raw honey)

Steps to Prepare:

1. Let the seeds soak in a bit of warm water for about 10 minutes until they form a thick paste.
2. Mix the soaked seeds gently with the plant gel and sweet syrup in a small bowl until smooth.
3. Spread the mixture evenly over clean skin, avoiding the eyes, and relax while it sits for around 20 minutes before rinsing off with cool water.

Suggested Usage:

Apply this gentle treatment every seven days to help keep your skin feeling soft and refreshed.

Important Cautions:

Always test a small amount on your inner arm first and wait a day to check for any skin irritation or sensitivity. Stop using if you notice redness or discomfort, and talk to a doctor if you have known allergies to plants or sweeteners.

Spicy Sweet Elixir for Smooth Digestion

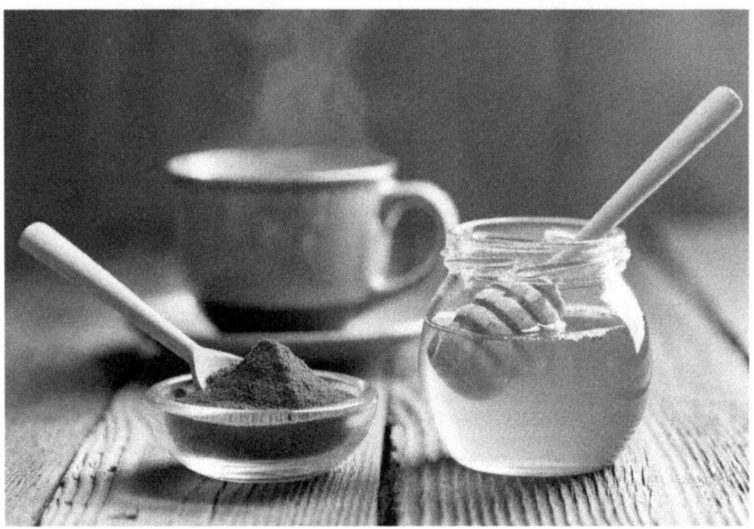

What You'll Need:

- A small dash (about 1/4 teaspoon) of cayenne pepper powder
- One generous spoonful (1 tablespoon) of pure, unprocessed honey
- A full cup of comfortably warm water

Steps to Prepare:

1. Pour the warm water into a mug or glass.
2. Sprinkle in the cayenne pepper powder and add the honey.
3. Mix everything together vigorously until the honey melts and the spice blends in evenly.

Suggested Usage:

Sip this tonic just before your main meals, aiming for two or three times per week to help keep your digestive system running smoothly.

Important Cautions:

Steer clear of this if you tend to have a delicate or easily irritated stomach, as the spice might cause discomfort. Always check with a healthcare provider if you have any gut-related conditions.

Lavender and Mint Soothing Soak

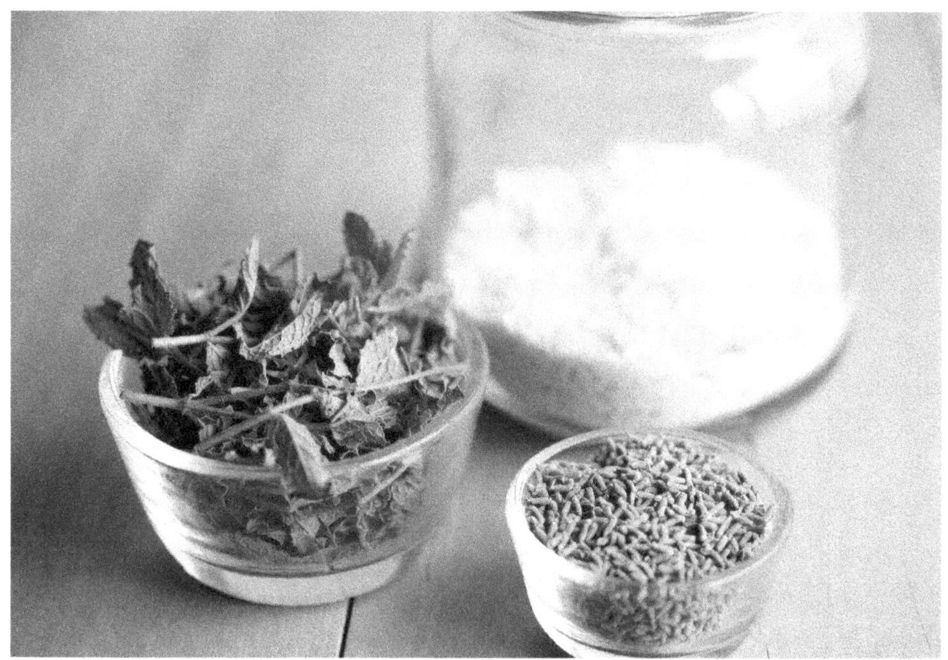

What You'll Need:

- 1/3 cup dried mint foliage
- 1/3 cup dried lavender blossoms
- 1.5 cups magnesium flakes

Steps to Prepare:

1. Mix the mint foliage, lavender blossoms, and magnesium flakes together in a clean container.
2. Pour the blend into a tub filled with comfortably hot water as it runs.
3. Stir gently to help everything dissolve and spread out.

Suggested Usage:

Add to your evening routine right before sleep to ease tension and promote calm.

Important Cautions:

Check for any sensitivity to herbs in the mint family or lavender beforehand; avoid if skin irritation occurs.

Golden Jojoba and Berry Seed Revitalizing Blend

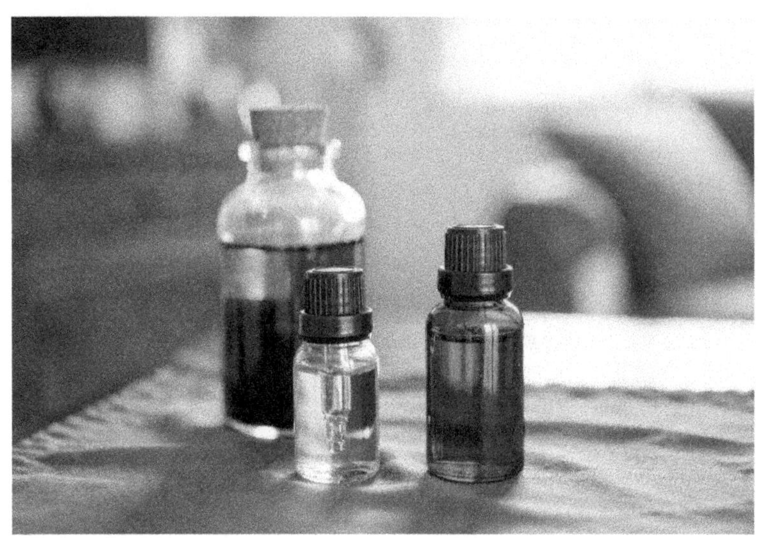

What You'll Need:

- 1 tablespoon golden jojoba carrier oil
- 1 tablespoon sea buckthorn berry oil
- 3 drops myrrh essential oil

Steps to Prepare:

1. Pour the carrier oils into a clean glass dropper bottle.
2. Add the essential oil drops and secure the cap.
3. Gently roll the bottle between your hands to blend everything together.

Suggested Usage:

Dab 2-3 drops onto your fingertips and massage lightly into freshly washed skin, focusing on dry or uneven areas.

Important Cautions:

Always do a small skin test on your inner arm first to check for any irritation, particularly if applying near sensitive spots like around the eyes.

Refreshing Cucumber Aloe Mist

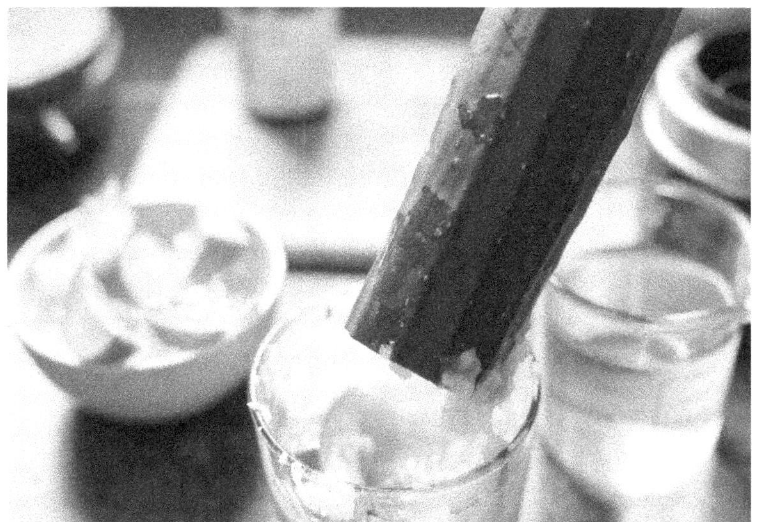

What You'll Need:

- One small fresh cucumber, blended into a smooth paste
- 1/4 cup pure aloe vera gel from the plant or store-bought
- 1/2 cup distilled water for better shelf life

Steps to Prepare:

1. Chop the cucumber into chunks and process it in a blender until it's completely smooth.
2. In a mixing bowl, stir the cucumber paste together with the aloe vera gel and distilled water until fully combined.
3. Transfer the mixture to a clean spray bottle using a funnel if needed.

Suggested Usage:

Lightly mist your face with the blend anytime your skin feels dry or needs a quick refresh during daily activities.

Important Cautions:

Do not spray directly into the eyes; if accidental contact happens, flush with cool water right away.

Herbal Defense Tonic

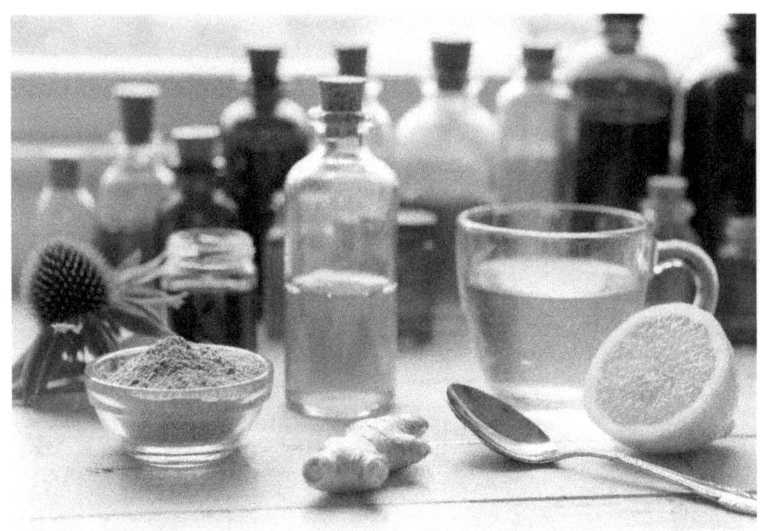

What You'll Need:

- 1 teaspoon of ground purple coneflower root
- A small piece (about half a thumb's length) of raw ginger root
- Juice from half a fresh lemon
- 1 spoonful of raw honey
- A quarter cup of hot water

Steps to Prepare:

1. Place the coneflower root and sliced ginger in a mug, then pour in the hot water and let it sit covered for about 15 minutes to draw out the flavors.
2. Pour the mixture through a fine mesh to remove the solids, then stir in the lemon juice and honey until everything blends smoothly.

Suggested Usage:

Take one small glass each morning when sniffles are going around to help support your body's natural defenses.

Important Cautions:

Skip this if you have a known sensitivity to plants in the daisy family, as it might cause discomfort.

Soothing Herbal Blend for Cough Comfort

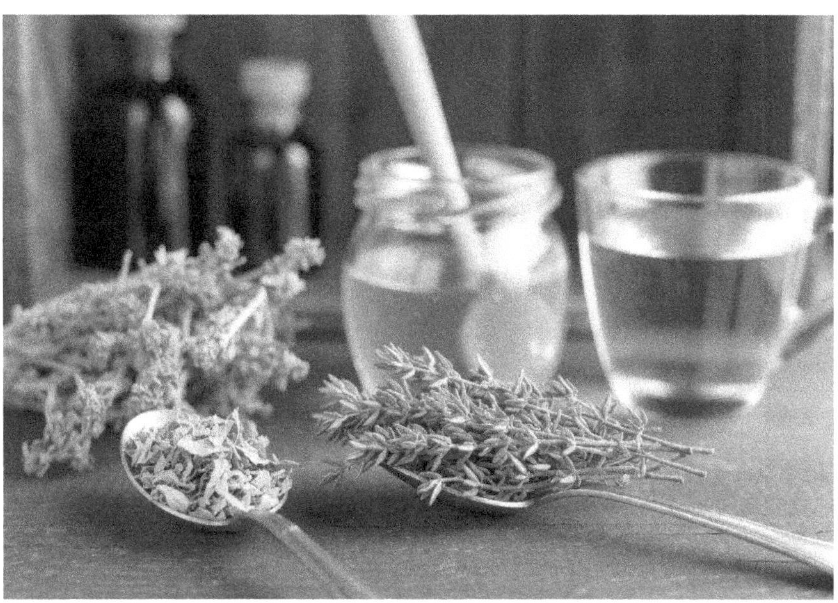

What You'll Need:

- 2 teaspoons of dried mullein foliage
- 2 teaspoons of dried thyme sprigs
- 3/4 cup of natural honey
- 1 1/4 cups of fresh water

Steps to Prepare:

1. Bring the water to a gentle boil in a small pot, then add the mullein and thyme.
2. Lower the heat and let the mixture simmer softly for about 10 minutes to draw out the helpful essences.
3. Remove from the stove, cover, and allow it to cool down to room temperature.
4. Filter out the plant material using a fine mesh or cloth, pressing lightly to get the liquid.
5. Stir in the honey until it's fully blended, then pour into a clean jar for storage in a cool spot.

Suggested Usage:

Spoon out 1 to 2 teaspoons as needed, up to three times throughout the day, to help ease throat irritation and support easier breathing.

Important Cautions:

Do not use it if you have a known sensitivity to herbs from the mint group, as this could cause reactions. Consult a healthcare provider before starting, especially if pregnant, nursing, or on medications.

Relaxing Herbal Blend for Stress Relief

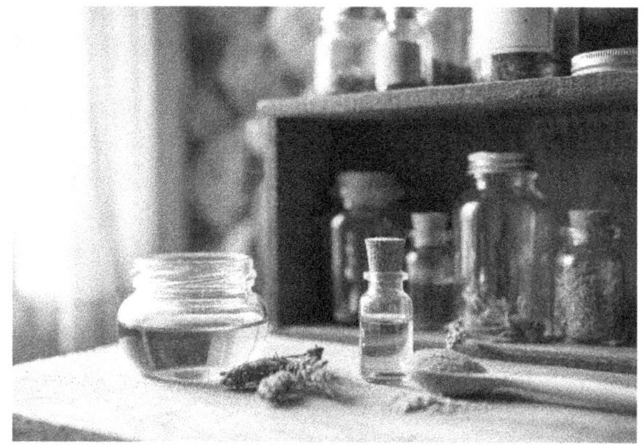

What You'll Need:

- 3 tablespoons of St. John's Wort infused oil
- 6 drops of lavender essential oil
- 2 teaspoons of sweet almond oil

Steps to Prepare:

1. Pour the St. John's Wort infused oil into a clean, dark-colored glass container.
2. Carefully add the drops of lavender essential oil and the sweet almond oil.
3. Secure the lid tightly and gently swirl the container to combine everything evenly.
4. Let the mixture rest in a cool spot for a full day to allow the scents and properties to meld together.

Suggested Usage:

Gently rub a small amount onto your wrists or the sides of your neck whenever tension builds up during the day.

Important Cautions:

Steer clear of this blend if you're currently using medications for mood support, as it could cause unwanted interactions. Always do a small skin test first to check for any irritation.

Citrus Herb Refreshing Infusion

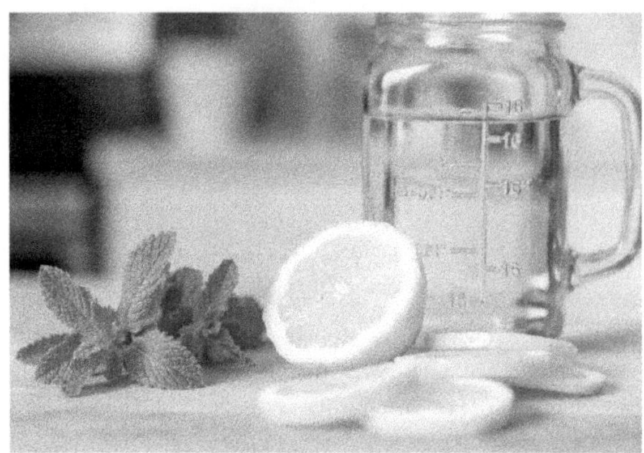

What You'll Need:

- 1 fresh lemon, cut into thin rounds
- A small bunch of fresh peppermint leaves (around 8 to 12)
- 16 ounces of filtered water

Steps to Prepare:

1. Place the lemon rounds and peppermint leaves in a clean glass container.
2. Pour the filtered water over the top.
3. Gently mash the leaves with the back of a spoon to help release their natural essences.
4. Cover the container and chill it in the fridge for about 60 minutes to allow the flavors to mix well.

Suggested Usage:

Enjoy sips of this cool drink spread out over your day to support your body's natural cleansing process.

Important Cautions:

This is usually safe for most people, but skip it if you're sensitive to citrus fruits. Always check with a healthcare provider if you have any health conditions or take medicines.

Soothing Mint and Tea Tree Mist for Skin Irritation

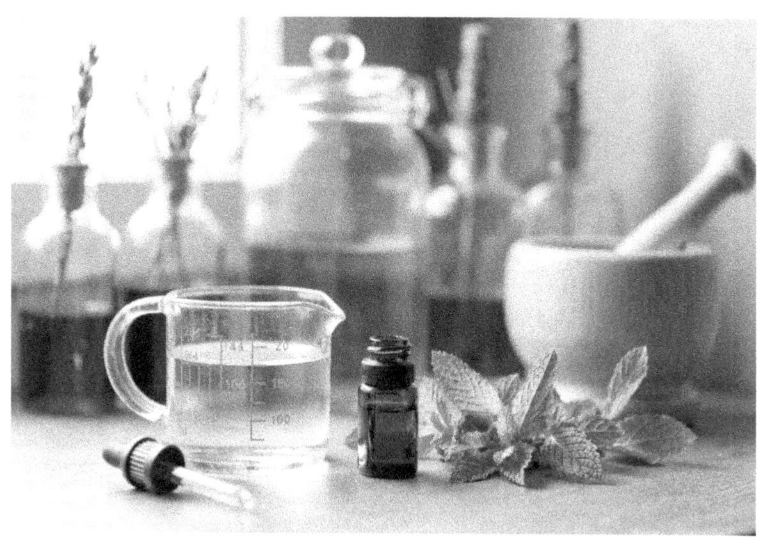

What You'll Need:

- 1/4 cup distilled water
- 8 drops of peppermint oil (from the mint plant)
- 12 drops of tea tree oil (a natural extract)

Steps to Prepare:

1. Pour the water into a small spray container.
2. Add the drops of peppermint and tea tree oils.
3. Secure the lid and give it a good swirl to blend everything together.

Suggested Usage:

Mist the blend lightly on areas of bothered skin whenever you feel the need for quick comfort. Always mix by shaking first to keep the oils evenly distributed.

Important Cautions:

Keep away from your face, especially the eye area, to prevent any stinging or discomfort. If you notice any unusual reaction on your skin, stop using it right away and rinse with cool water.

Ginger and Clove Soothing Blend for Lip Blisters

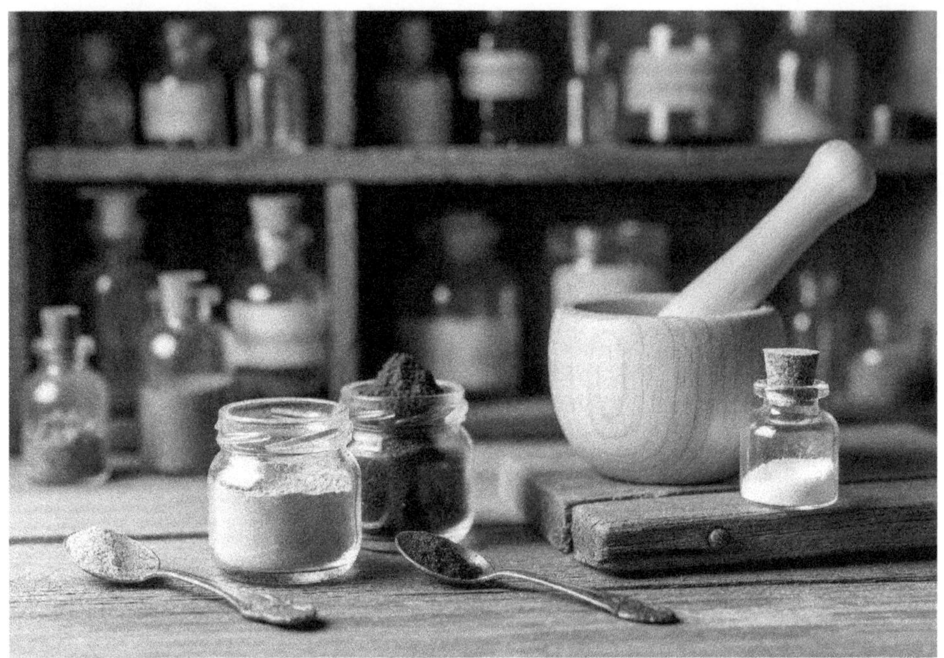

What You'll Need:

- 1/2 teaspoon powdered ginger
- 1/4 teaspoon powdered cloves
- 1 tablespoon softened coconut oil

Steps to Prepare:

1. Blend the powdered ginger and cloves together in a small dish.
2. Add the coconut oil and stir well until it turns into a smooth mixture.
3. Dab a small amount directly on the spot.

Suggested Usage:

Gently apply two or three times each day until the area feels better.

Important Cautions:

Skip this if the skin is cut or raw to prevent irritation.

Silymarin Seed Infusion for Gentle Liver Cleanse

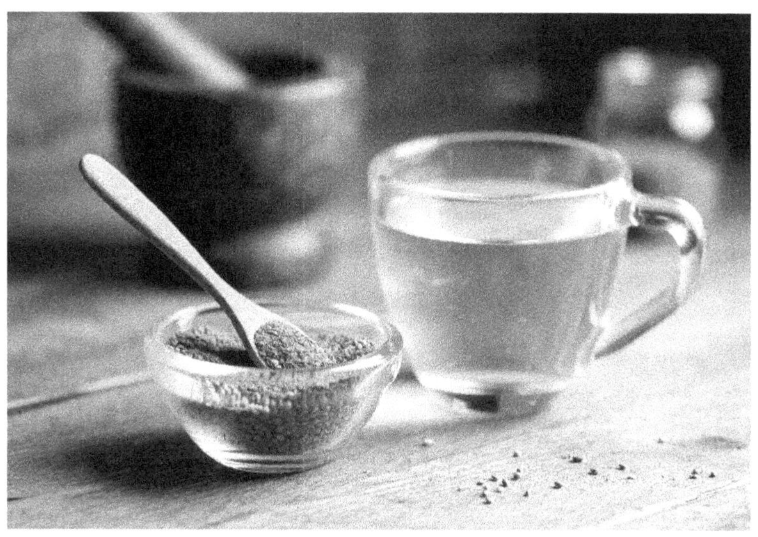

What You'll Need:

- 1 teaspoon of crushed silymarin seeds (from the milk thistle plant)
- 1 cup of freshly boiled water

Steps to Prepare:

1. Place the crushed seeds into a mug or teapot.
2. Pour the boiling water over them and let it sit covered for about 10 minutes to draw out the beneficial compounds.
3. Filter out the seeds using a fine mesh strainer, then sip the warm liquid.

Suggested Usage:

Enjoy one serving each day as part of your routine to help your body naturally flush out toxins and maintain liver health.

Important Cautions:

Talk to your healthcare provider before starting if you're taking any prescriptions related to liver conditions, as interactions could occur.

Soothing Belly Comfort Infusion

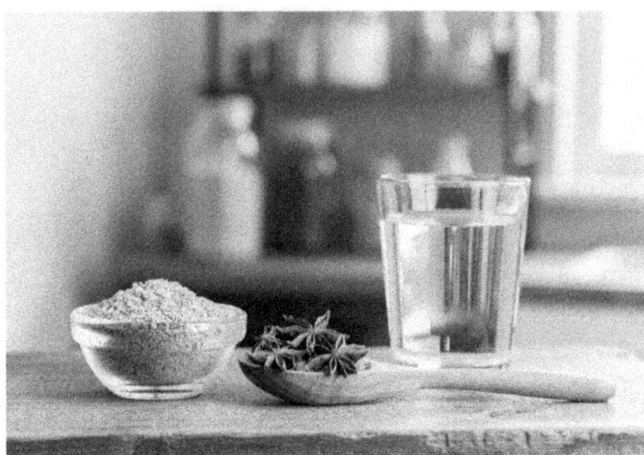

What You'll Need:

- 1 teaspoon crushed anise seeds (for a mild, sweet flavor that eases bloating)
- 1 teaspoon dried sweet root pieces (to calm the stomach lining)
- 1 cup fresh water

Steps to Prepare:

1. Pour the water into a small saucepan and heat it until it starts to bubble.
2. Stir in the anise seeds and sweet root pieces.
3. Lower the heat and let the mix gently simmer for about 5 minutes to draw out the natural essences.
4. Pour through a fine mesh strainer into your favorite mug, discarding the solids.

Suggested Usage:

Enjoy a warm cup once or twice daily, especially after meals, to promote smooth digestion and reduce discomfort.

Important Cautions:

Skip this if you deal with elevated blood pressure, since sweet root might influence it. Always check with a doctor if you're unsure or have health conditions.

Herbal Scalp Nourishment Blend

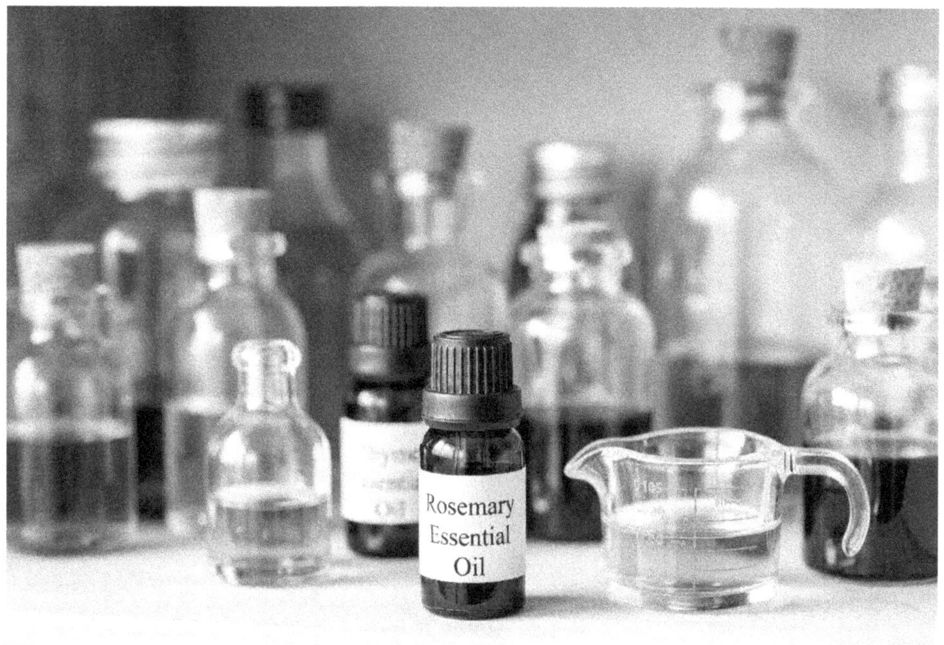

What You'll Need:

- 1 tablespoon rosemary essential oil
- 1 tablespoon thyme essential oil
- 2 tablespoons olive oil (as a gentle base)

Steps to Prepare:

1. Pour the olive oil into a small container.
2. Add the rosemary and thyme essential oils, then stir gently until fully mixed.

Suggested Usage:

Gently rub the mixture onto your scalp using your fingertips, then let it sit for about 30 minutes before rinsing with mild shampoo.

Important Cautions:

Do not use it if you are expecting a baby. Always test a small amount on your skin first to check for any irritation.

Energizing Morning Infusion

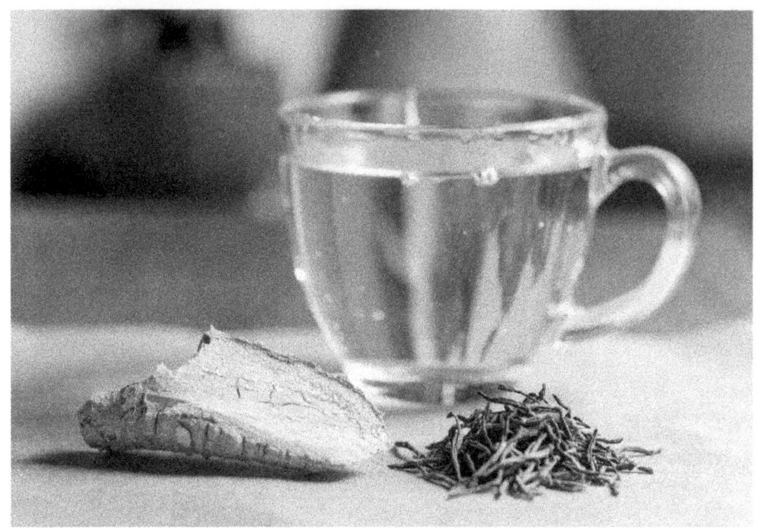

What You'll Need:

- A small slice of dried ginseng root (about 1 teaspoon when chopped)
- 1 teaspoon of loose green tea leaves
- 1 cup of freshly boiled water

Steps to Prepare:

1. Place the ginseng slice and green tea leaves into a mug or teapot.
2. Pour the hot water over them and let the mixture sit covered for about 6 minutes to allow the flavors and benefits to blend.
3. Use a fine mesh strainer to separate the liquid from the solids, then enjoy the warm brew.

Suggested Usage:

Sip this infusion right after waking up to help invigorate your day and support natural alertness.

Important Cautions:

Steer clear of this if you have trouble with stimulants, such as feeling jittery from coffee. Always check with a healthcare provider if you have health conditions or take medications.

Rose and Hibiscus Radiance Facial Blend

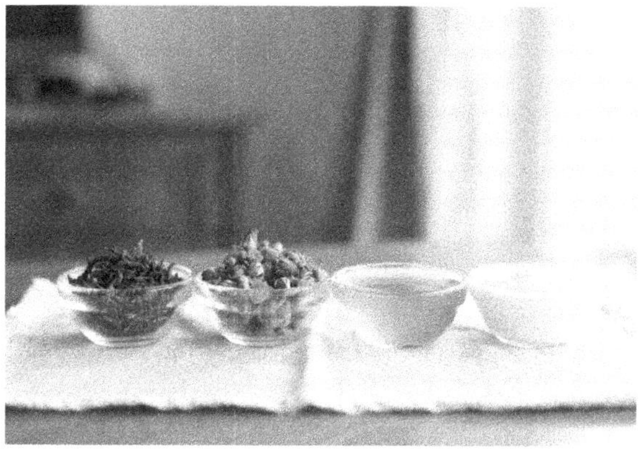

What You'll Need:

- 1 tablespoon of crushed hibiscus flowers (dried)
- 1 tablespoon of rose buds (dried)
- 1 tablespoon of natural honey
- 1 tablespoon of plain yogurt

Steps to Prepare:

1. Crush the hibiscus flowers and rose buds into small bits using a mortar and pestle or a blender.
2. Combine the crushed bits with the honey and yogurt in a small bowl, stirring until it forms a smooth mixture.
3. Spread the mixture evenly over your clean face, avoiding the eye area, and relax for about 15 minutes before rinsing off with warm water.

Suggested Usage:

Apply this blend once every seven days to help enhance your skin's natural glow and even tone.

Important Cautions:

Always do a small patch test on your inner arm 24 hours before full use to check for any skin reactions.

Soothing Spice Blend for Swelling Relief

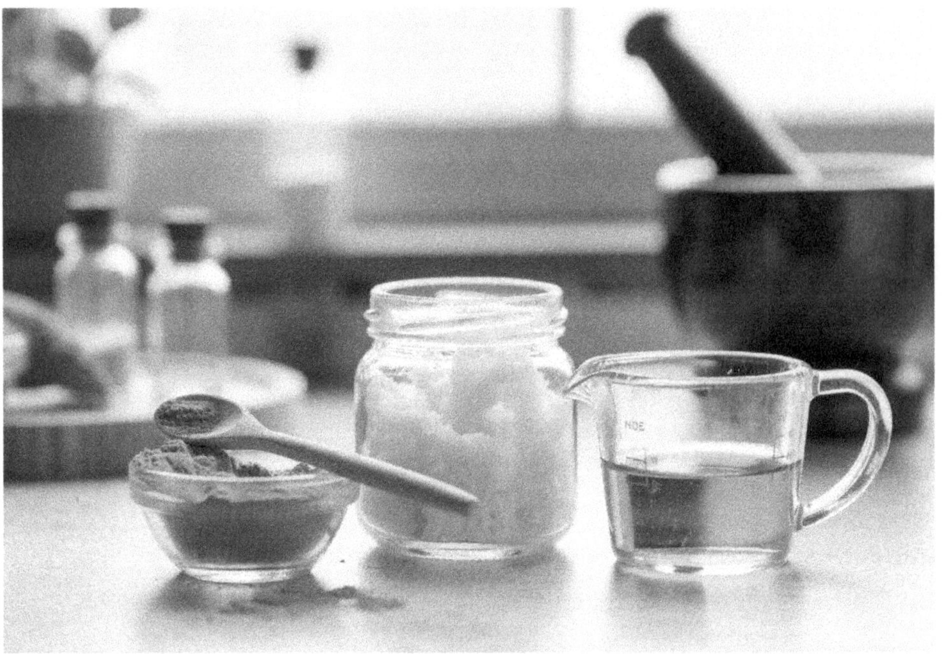

What You'll Need:

- 2 teaspoons ground turmeric
- 1 teaspoon freshly grated ginger root
- 1 tablespoon olive oil

Steps to Prepare:

1. Peel and finely grate the ginger root.
2. In a small bowl, stir the grated ginger together with the turmeric.
3. Gradually add the olive oil, mixing until you get a smooth, spreadable mixture.

Suggested Usage:

Gently spread a thin layer on sore or puffy spots up to two times each day to help ease discomfort.

Important Cautions:

Steer clear if the skin has any open cuts or scrapes.

Warming Spice Infusion for Cold Relief

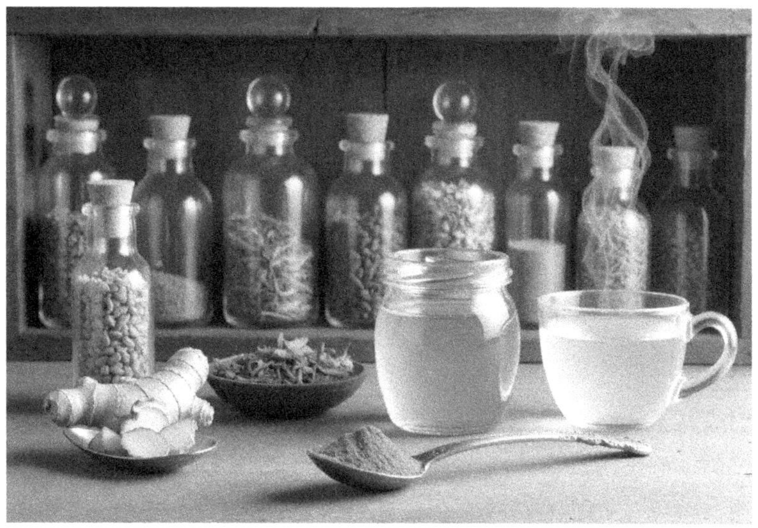

What You'll Need:

- 2 teaspoons freshly chopped ginger root
- 1/2 teaspoon ground cinnamon
- 1 teaspoon raw honey
- 8 ounces boiling water

Steps to Prepare:

1. Place the chopped ginger and ground cinnamon into a heat-safe mug.
2. Pour the boiling water over the spices and cover the mug to keep the heat in.
3. Allow it to steep for about 8 minutes to draw out the flavors.
4. Stir in the honey until it dissolves completely.

Suggested Usage:

Sip this warm drink once or twice each day to help ease stuffiness and discomfort from a cold.

Important Cautions:

Check with your healthcare provider before using if you're on medications that affect blood clotting.

Boosting Defense Syrup with Coneflower and Dark Berries

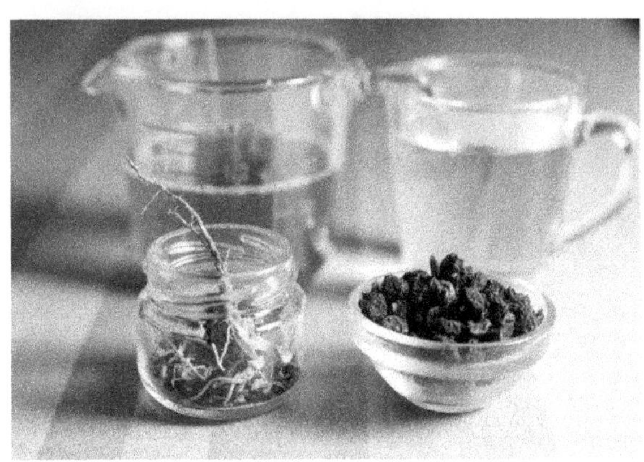

What You'll Need:

- 1 tablespoon dried coneflower root (echinacea)
- 1 tablespoon dried dark berries (elderberries)
- 1/2 cup natural sweetener (honey)
- 1 cup clean water

Steps to Prepare:

1. Pour the water into a small saucepan and add the coneflower root along with the dark berries.
2. Heat the mixture until it starts bubbling lightly, then lower the flame and let it cook slowly for 15 to 25 minutes to draw out the helpful elements.
3. Take it off the stove, filter away the plant pieces using a fine mesh or cloth, and blend in the sweetener while it's still warm for easy mixing.

Suggested Usage:

Swallow one spoonful every day as a simple way to help your body stay strong against everyday challenges.

Important Cautions:

Skip this if you're expecting a baby or nursing, as it might not be suitable during those times.

Soothing Aloe Cucumber Blend for Sun Relief

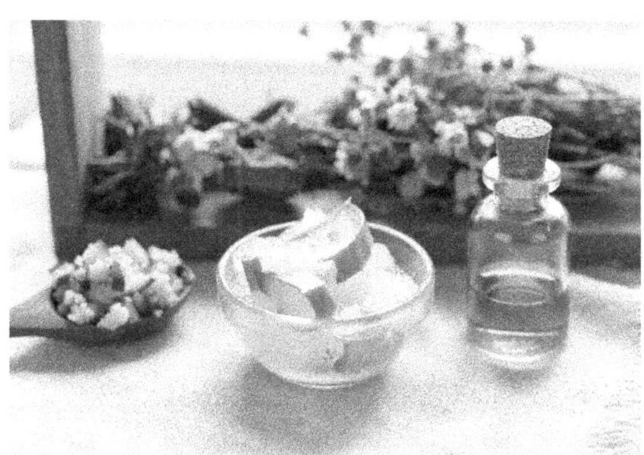

What You'll Need:

- 3 tablespoons fresh aloe vera gel (from the plant or store-bought pure gel)
- 2 tablespoons fresh cucumber puree (blend a small cucumber section and strain)
- 1 teaspoon olive oil

Steps to Prepare:

1. Scoop the aloe vera gel into a small bowl.
2. Blend a piece of cucumber until smooth, then strain to collect the clear liquid.
3. Stir the cucumber liquid and olive oil into the aloe until it forms a smooth mixture.
4. Store in a clean jar in the fridge for up to a week.

Suggested Usage:

Gently spread a thin layer on red or tender skin areas after sun exposure. Reapply every few hours or when the skin feels warm again.

Important Cautions:

Apply only to unbroken skin. Stop using if any redness or itching occurs, and rinse off right away. Keep away from eyes and mouth.

Relaxing Herb Infusion for Peaceful Nights

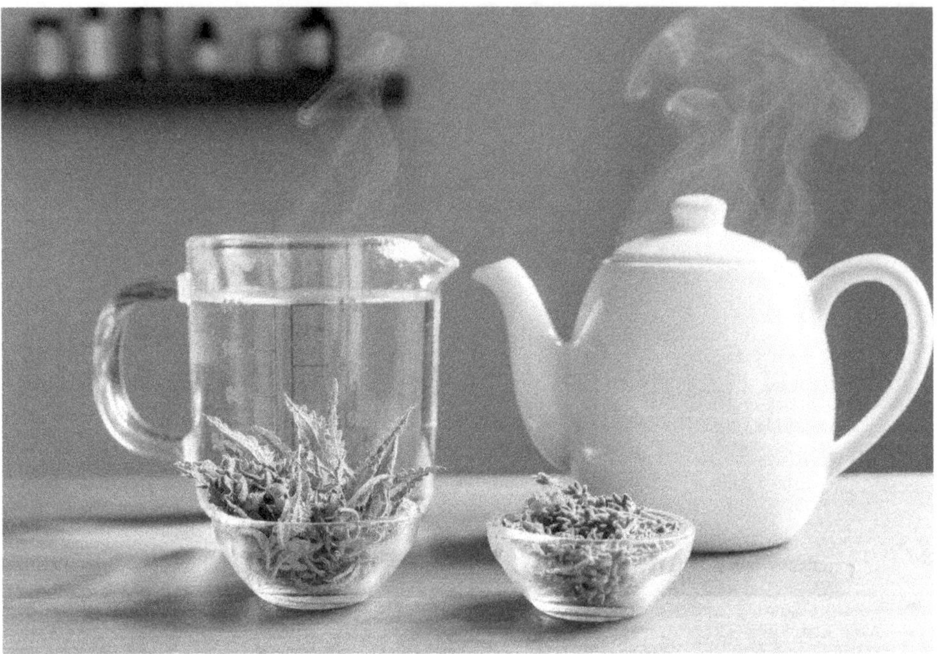

What You'll Need:

- 1 teaspoon of dried lemon balm leaves
- 1 teaspoon of lavender blossoms
- 8 ounces of freshly boiled water

Steps to Prepare:

1. Combine the lemon balm and lavender in a mug or infuser.
2. Add the boiling water and cover to keep the warmth in.
3. Allow the mixture to infuse for 8 to 12 minutes.
4. Remove the herbs by straining, then sip slowly.

Suggested Usage:

Enjoy this brew about half an hour before turning in for the night to encourage deeper relaxation and improved sleep quality.

Important Cautions:

Skip this if you're expecting a baby, as it may not be suitable during that time.

Soothing Spice Blend for Muscle Discomfort

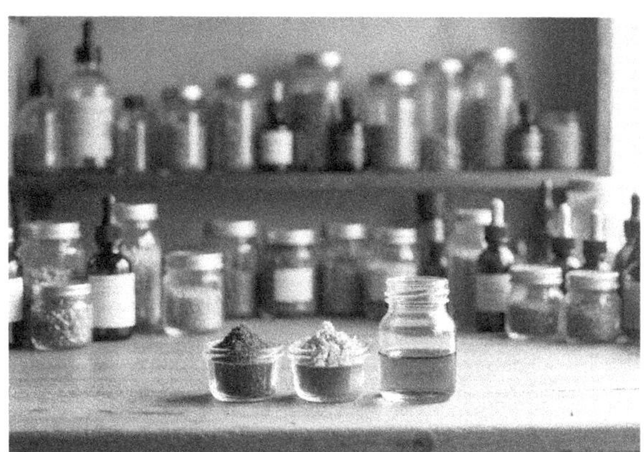

What You'll Need:

- 1 tablespoon finely ground red pepper flakes
- 1 tablespoon concentrated ginger essence
- 2 tablespoons mild carrier oil, such as from olives

Steps to Prepare:

1. Combine the ground red pepper flakes and ginger essence into the carrier oil in a small container.
2. Stir thoroughly until everything blends smoothly, creating a warming mixture ready for application.
3. Gently rub the blend onto areas of muscle tension for a comforting effect.

Suggested Usage:

Rub a small amount onto the affected spots up to three times daily to help ease aches and promote relaxation.

Important Cautions:

Keep away from sensitive areas like your eyes or any delicate skin linings to prevent irritation. Test on a small patch of skin first if you're new to these ingredients.

Brain Boost Herbal Infusion

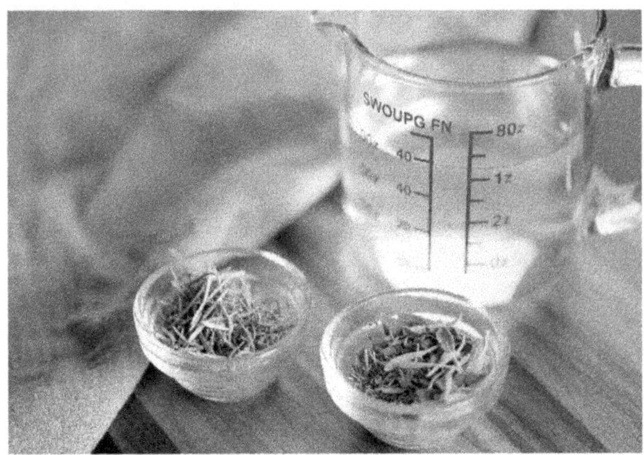

What You'll Need:

- 2 teaspoons dried rosemary sprigs
- 1 teaspoon dried sage foliage
- 8 ounces boiling water

Steps to Prepare:

1. Place the rosemary and sage in a mug or teapot.
2. Pour the boiling water over the herbs and cover to keep the heat in.
3. Allow the mixture to infuse for about 15 minutes to draw out the natural essences.
4. Use a fine mesh strainer to separate the liquid from the plant material, then enjoy the warm brew.

Suggested Usage:

Sip one serving each morning to help support mental clarity and focus throughout your day.

Important Cautions:

Do not use this if you are expecting a baby, as it may not be suitable during pregnancy. Consult a healthcare provider if you have any health conditions or take medications.

Mint and Eucalyptus Vapor Inhalation for Clear Airways

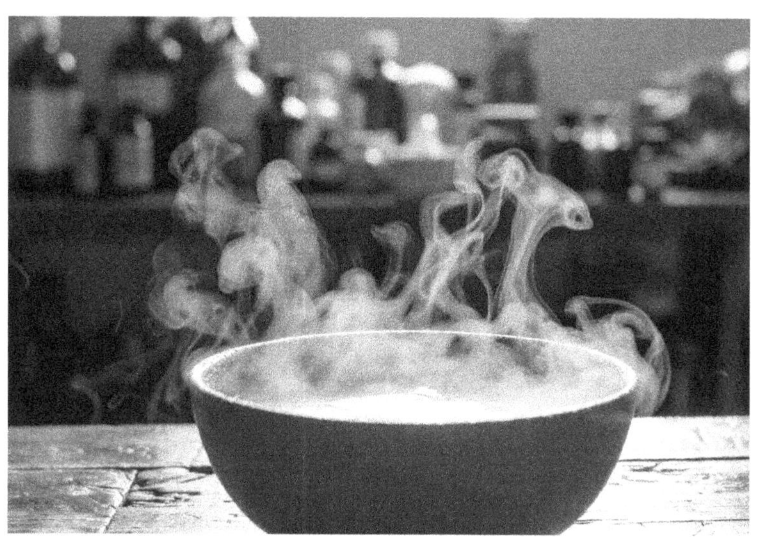

What You'll Need:

- 4-6 drops of peppermint essential oil
- 4-6 drops of eucalyptus essential oil
- A large bowl filled with steaming hot water

Steps to Prepare:

1. Pour the essential oils directly into the bowl of hot water.
2. Position your face over the bowl, keeping a safe distance to avoid burns, and breathe in the rising vapors deeply for about 10 minutes.

Suggested Usage:

Try this inhalation method two to three times a day to help ease stuffy sinuses and promote comfortable breathing.

Important Cautions:

Avoid using this around infants or young children, as the strong aromas could be too intense for them.

Calming Oat and Chamomile Blend for Delicate Skin

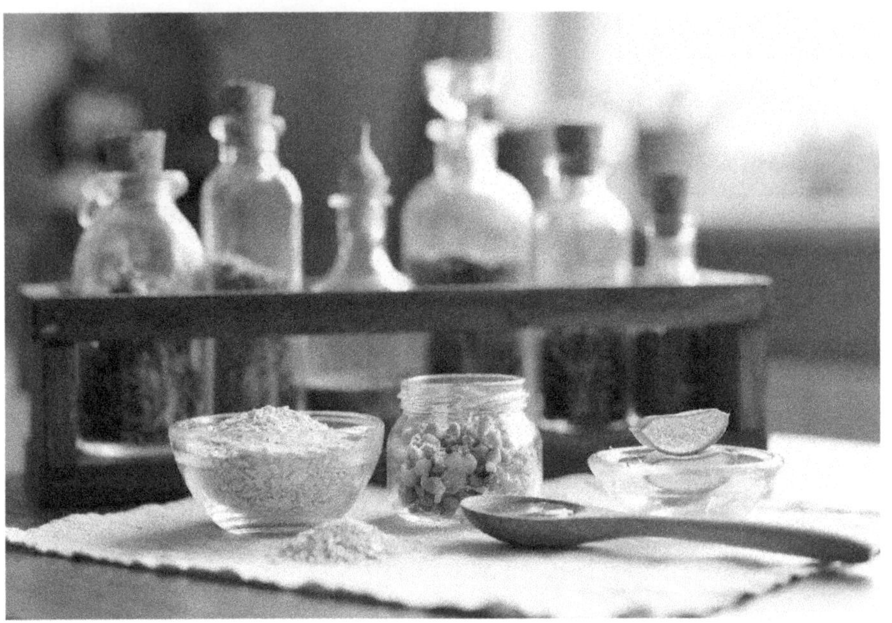

What You'll Need:

- 1 tablespoon of finely ground oats
- 1 tablespoon of dried chamomile blossoms
- 1 tablespoon of pure honey
- 1 tablespoon of fresh aloe vera gel

Steps to Prepare:

1. Crush the chamomile blossoms into small pieces using a mortar and pestle or a clean coffee grinder.
2. In a small bowl, stir the crushed chamomile together with the ground oats.
3. Add the honey and aloe vera gel, mixing everything until it forms a thick, even paste.

Suggested Usage:

Gently spread the paste over your clean face, avoiding the eyes. Let it sit for about 10 to 15 minutes while you relax, then rinse off with lukewarm water. Try this once every seven days to help calm and comfort touchy skin.

Before full use, apply a small amount to the inside of your wrist and wait 24 hours to check for any skin irritation or allergic response. Stop using if redness or discomfort occurs.

Soothing Ginger Infusion for Throat Ease

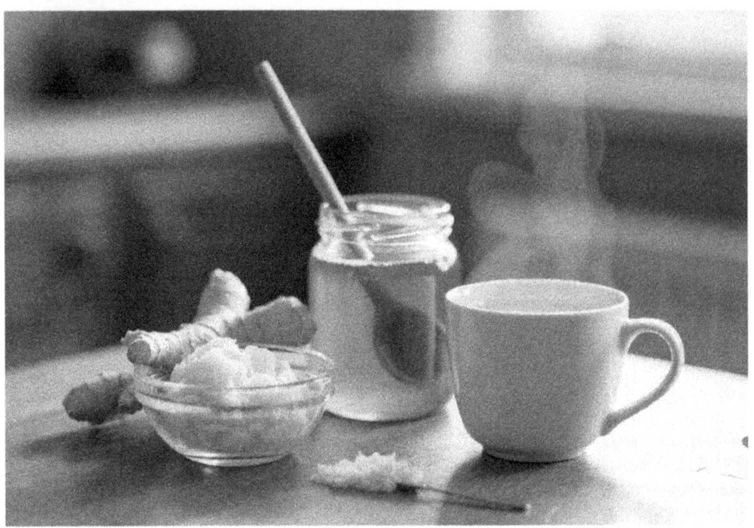

What You'll Need:

- 1 tablespoon fresh ginger root, peeled and minced
- 1 tablespoon pure honey
- 1 cup hot water (not boiling)

Steps to Prepare:

1. Place the minced ginger in a cup or mug.
2. Add the honey on top.
3. Pour the hot water over the mixture and stir gently until the honey fully melts in.
4. Allow it to steep for 5 minutes to let the flavors blend, then enjoy while warm.

Suggested Usage:

Sip on this infusion two to three times each day to help calm an uncomfortable throat.

Important Cautions:

Do not offer this to babies under one year of age, as honey can pose a health risk for them.

Soothing Herbal Balm for Congestion Ease

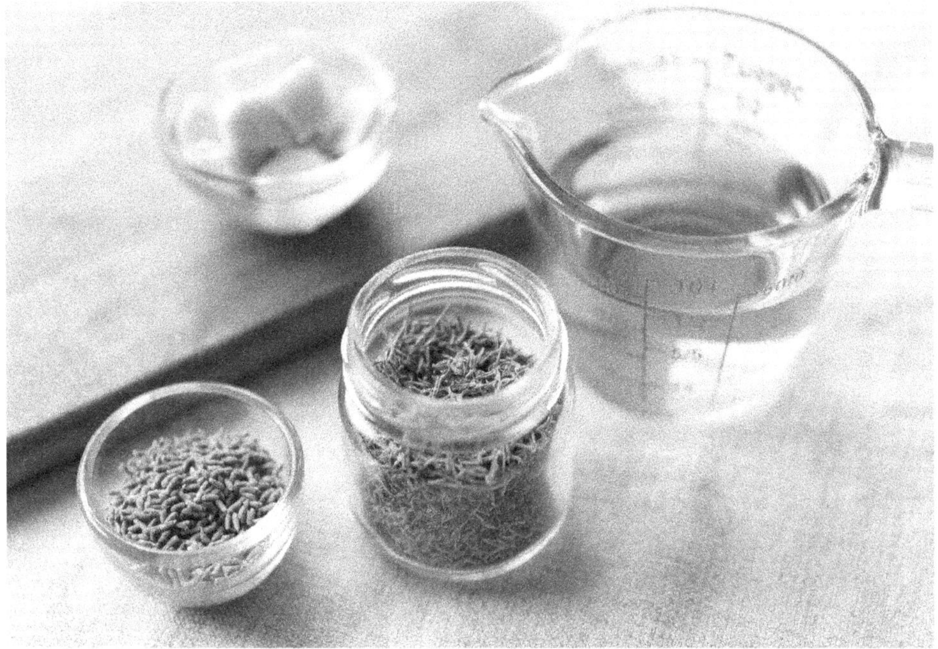

What You'll Need:

- 2 tablespoons dried thyme leaves
- 2 tablespoons dried lavender buds
- 1/2 cup olive oil (as a gentle base)
- 1 tablespoon beeswax pastilles

Steps to Prepare:

1. Place the olive oil in a double boiler over low heat, then stir in the thyme leaves and lavender buds. Allow the mixture to warm gently for 45 minutes, stirring occasionally to draw out the natural properties.
2. Take the pot off the heat and filter the oil through a clean cloth or fine strainer to remove the plant material.
3. In a separate small pan, melt the beeswax over low heat until fully liquid, then blend it into the warm, herb-infused oil until smooth.
4. Pour the combined mixture into a small jar or tin and let it set at room temperature until firm.

Suggested Usage:

Gently massage a pea-sized amount onto the upper chest area to help soothe discomfort from stuffiness or chills.

Perform a small skin test by applying a tiny bit to your inner arm and waiting 24 hours to watch for any irritation or sensitivity. Avoid use if you notice redness or discomfort. Consult a healthcare provider if symptoms persist or if you're pregnant, nursing, or have underlying health conditions.

Refreshing Green Citrus Cleanse Blend

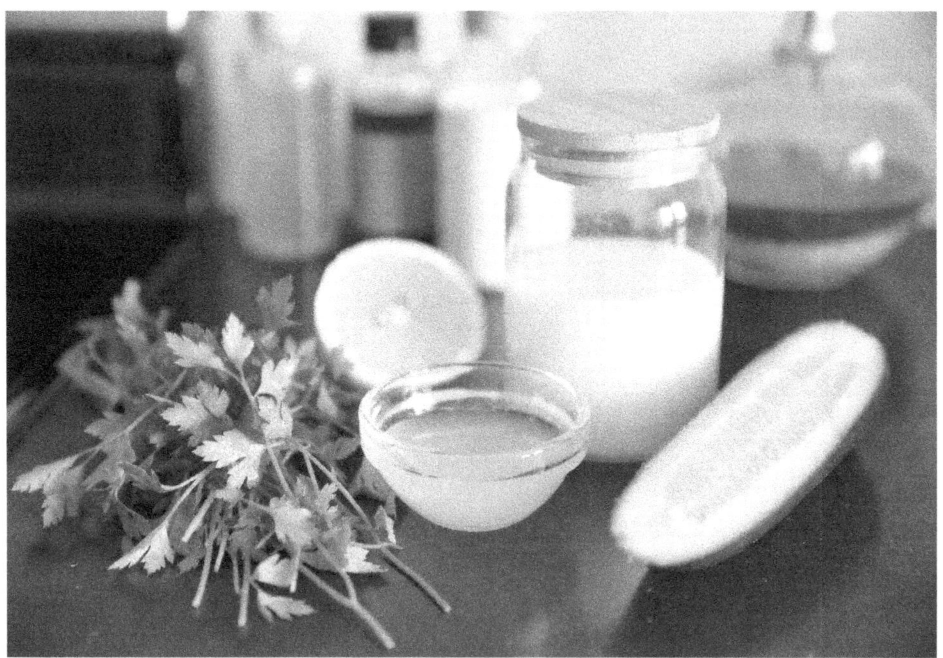

What You'll Need:

- A small bunch of fresh parsley (about 1/4 cup)
- Juice squeezed from half a lemon
- 1 cup of coconut liquid
- Half a cucumber, sliced

Steps to Prepare:

1. Add the parsley, lemon juice, coconut liquid, and cucumber pieces into a blender.
2. Mix on high speed until everything combines into a silky texture.

Suggested Usage:

Sip this beverage right after you wake up to support your body's natural cleansing process.

Important Cautions:

Avoid this if you know you react badly to parsley.

Soothing Root Blend for Queasy Moments

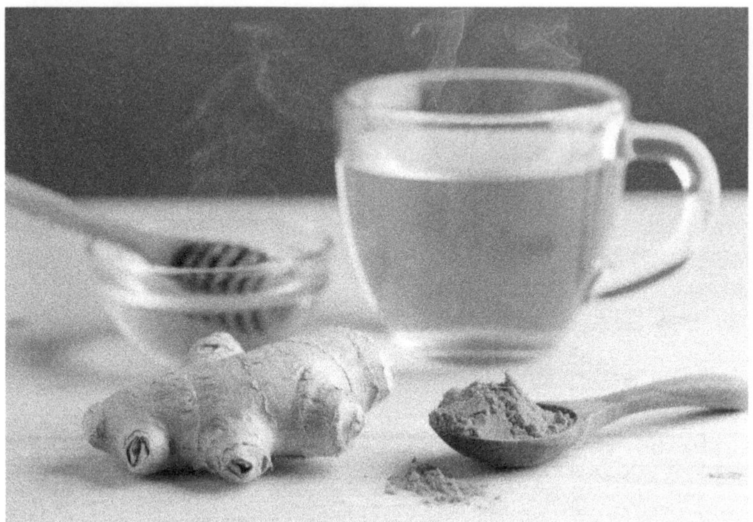

What You'll Need:

- 1 small piece of fresh ginger (about the size of your thumb)
- 1/4 teaspoon ground turmeric
- 1 teaspoon natural sweetener like honey
- 1 cup of comfortably hot water

Steps to Prepare:

1. Peel the ginger and chop it into small bits to release its juices.
2. Combine the chopped ginger with the turmeric in a cup.
3. Pour the hot water over the mixture and let it sit for 5 minutes to infuse.
4. Mix in the sweetener until it fully dissolves, then strain out the solids if you prefer a smoother drink.

Suggested Usage:

Sip the blend slowly whenever your stomach feels unsettled, up to twice a day.

Important Cautions:

Skip this if you're expecting a baby, as it might not suit everyone in that stage. Check with a healthcare provider if you have any ongoing gut or liver concerns.

Lavender and Orange Revitalizing Foot Bath

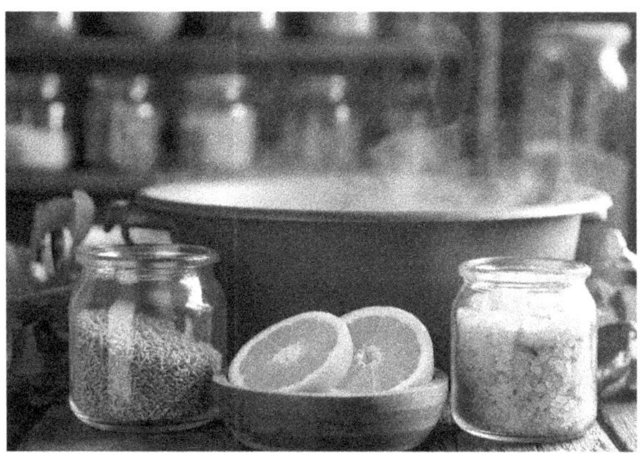

What You'll Need:

- 1/3 cup dried lavender buds
- 1 fresh orange, cut into thin rounds
- 3/4 cup sea salt
- A large basin filled with comfortably hot water

Steps to Prepare:

1. Pour the hot water into your basin.
2. Sprinkle in the lavender buds, drop in the orange rounds, and stir in the sea salt until it starts to dissolve.
3. Allow the mixture to sit for about 5 minutes so the scents and properties can blend together.

Suggested Usage:

Ideal for unwinding after a long day while helping your body feel refreshed and purified. Soak your feet in the bath for 20-25 minutes, then pat dry.

Important Cautions:

Do not use it if your skin is prone to irritation or if you have any open cuts on your feet. Test a small area first if unsure.

Relaxing Lavender-Chamomile Bedtime Mist

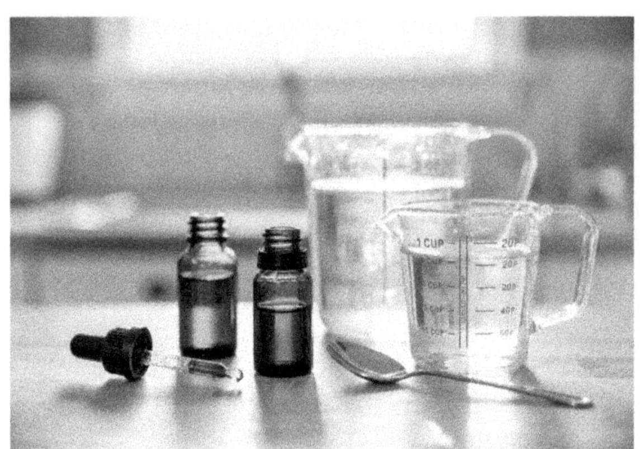

What You'll Need:

- 8 drops lavender essential oil
- 12 drops chamomile essential oil
- 1 cup distilled water
- 2 teaspoons vodka (or alcohol-free alternative like vegetable glycerin)

Steps to Prepare:

1. Start by adding the distilled water to a clean glass spray bottle.
2. Drop in the lavender and chamomile essential oils carefully.
3. Stir in the vodka to help the oils blend evenly with the water.
4. Cap the bottle tightly and give it a good shake for about 30 seconds to combine everything.

Suggested Usage:

Spray a gentle mist over your sheets or pillowcase each evening as part of your wind-down routine to encourage peaceful rest.

Important Cautions:

Do not spray near your face, especially avoiding contact with eyes or sensitive skin areas. Test on a small fabric patch first to check for staining.

Soothing Aromatic Vapor for Stuffy Nose Ease

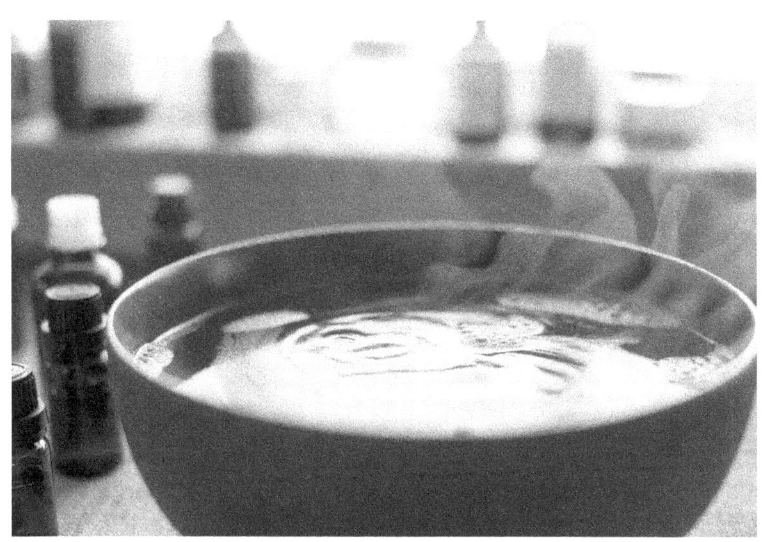

What You'll Need:

- 4 drops of peppermint essential oil
- 4 drops of eucalyptus essential oil
- A large bowl filled with steaming hot water

Steps to Prepare:

1. Fill a big bowl with freshly boiled water.
2. Carefully mix in the peppermint and eucalyptus oils.
3. Place a towel over your head to trap the rising mist, then lean close to the bowl.

Suggested Usage:

Breathe in the warm vapors slowly and steadily for around 8 to 12 minutes whenever your sinuses feel clogged.

Important Cautions:

Keep this away from babies and young kids, as the strong aromas could be too much for them.

Soothing Spice and Sweetener Mix for Cough Comfort

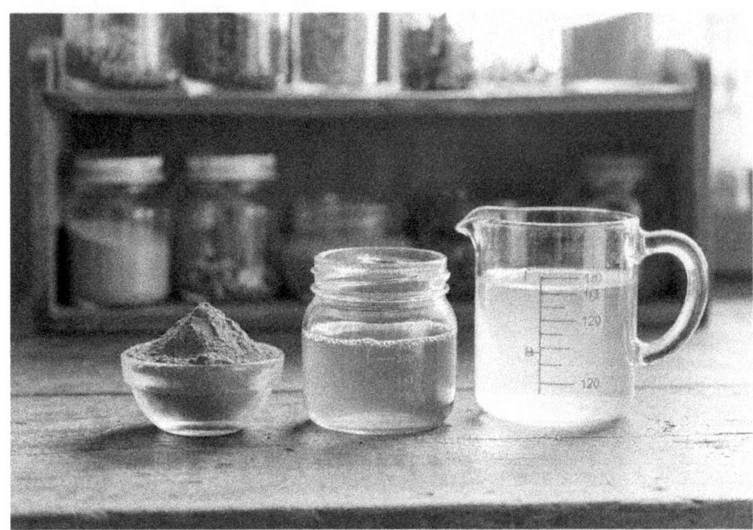

What You'll Need:

- 1 teaspoon powdered cinnamon
- 3 tablespoons pure honey
- 1/3 cup lukewarm water

Steps to Prepare:

1. Start by warming the water just enough so it's comfortable to touch.
2. Blend the honey into the water first, mixing steadily to combine them.
3. Gradually add the cinnamon while continuing to stir, ensuring the mixture becomes smooth without clumps.

Suggested Usage:

Spoon out 1 small portion periodically during the day to help ease discomfort.

Important Cautions:

Avoid administering to babies less than 12 months old, as honey can pose health risks for them.

Soothing Stomach Blend with Vinegar and Nectar

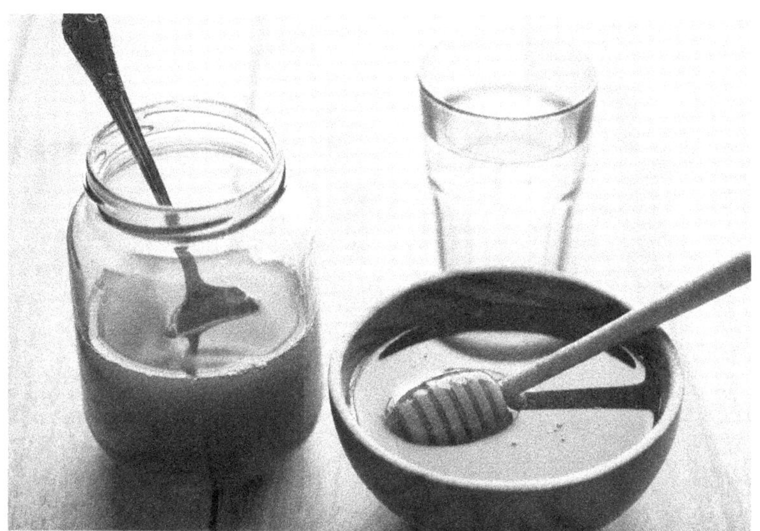

What You'll Need:

- One large spoon of unfiltered apple cider vinegar
- One large spoon of pure, raw honey
- Eight ounces of lukewarm water

Steps to Prepare:

1. Pour the lukewarm water into a glass or mug.
2. Stir in the apple cider vinegar followed by the honey until everything blends smoothly.
3. Give it a final mix to ensure it's well combined.

Suggested Usage:

Enjoy this drink each day, ideally right before eating, to help ease your tummy and promote smooth processing of food.

Important Cautions:

Skip this if your stomach is empty and you often deal with heartburn or similar discomfort, as it might make things worse.

Natural Blemish Reducer with Nigella Oil and Citrus

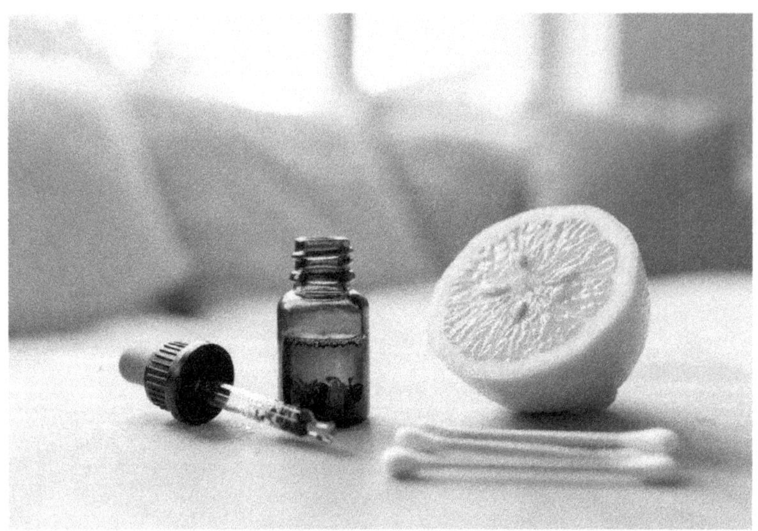

What You'll Need:

- 1 tablespoon nigella seed oil (also known as black seed oil)
- Fresh juice from half a lemon (roughly 1 tablespoon)
- A few clean cotton swabs

Steps to Prepare:

1. Squeeze the juice from half a lemon into a small bowl.
2. Pour in the nigella seed oil and whisk together until evenly combined.
3. Dip a cotton swab into the blend to pick up a small amount.

Suggested Usage:

Gently press the soaked swab onto blemishes or breakout areas once each day, after washing your face.

Important Cautions:

Do a small skin test on your wrist first to make sure there's no irritation. Lemon juice can increase skin's sensitivity to sunlight, so use this in the evening and wear sunscreen during the day.

Immune Boosting Blend in Easy Capsules

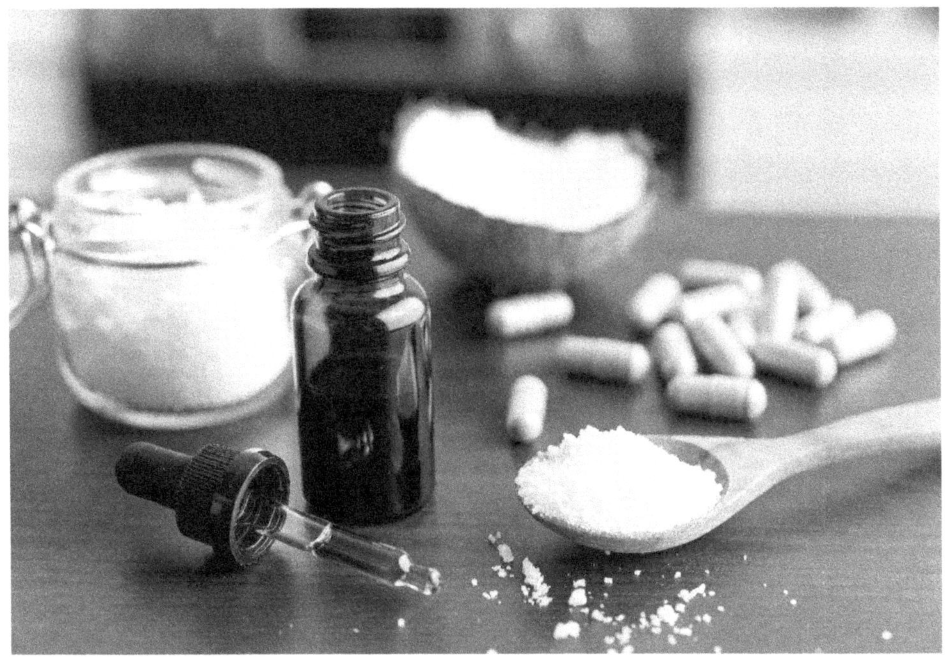

What You'll Need:

- Just one drop of essential oil from oregano
- A single tablespoon of pure coconut oil
- Some empty gelatin or veggie capsules

Steps to Prepare:

1. Gently stir the oregano essential oil into the coconut oil until they're fully blended together.
2. Carefully spoon or pipette the combined oils into the empty capsules, sealing them shut.

Suggested Usage:

Swallow one capsule each day to help strengthen your body's natural defenses against everyday bugs.

Important Cautions:

Oregano essential oil packs a strong punch, so handle it with care and consider consulting a health expert if you're new to it or have sensitivities.

Nutty Sweet Facial Reviver

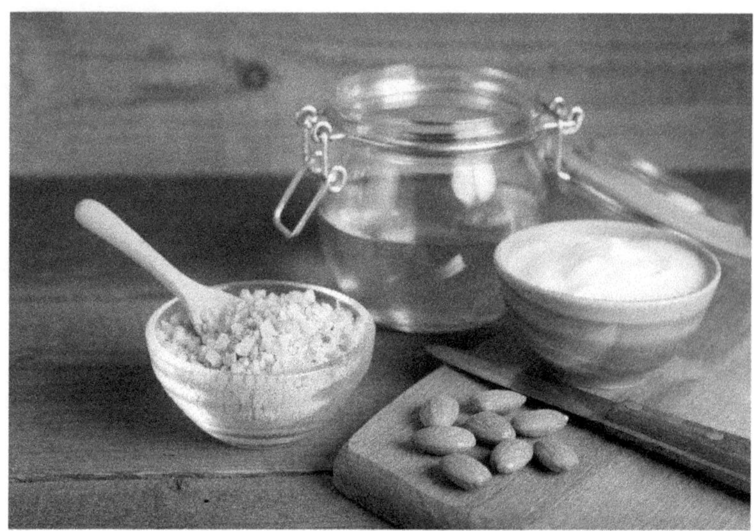

What You'll Need:

- 1 tablespoon finely crushed nuts (like almonds)
- 1 tablespoon natural sweetener (such as honey)
- 1 tablespoon smooth dairy base (plain yogurt works well)

Steps to Prepare:

1. Combine the crushed nuts, sweetener, and dairy base in a small bowl.
2. Stir everything together until it forms a thick, spreadable mixture.
3. Let the blend rest for a couple of minutes to allow the textures to meld.

Suggested Usage:

Apply a thin layer to clean skin, avoiding the eyes, and leave it on for about 10-15 minutes before rinsing with warm water. Try this once every seven days to help promote a softer, more refreshed complexion.

Important Cautions:

Always do a small patch test on your inner arm first to check for any skin sensitivity or reactions. If you notice redness or itching, stop using it right away. Consult a doctor if you have nut allergies or sensitive skin conditions.

Soothing Mint and Eucalyptus Skin Calmer

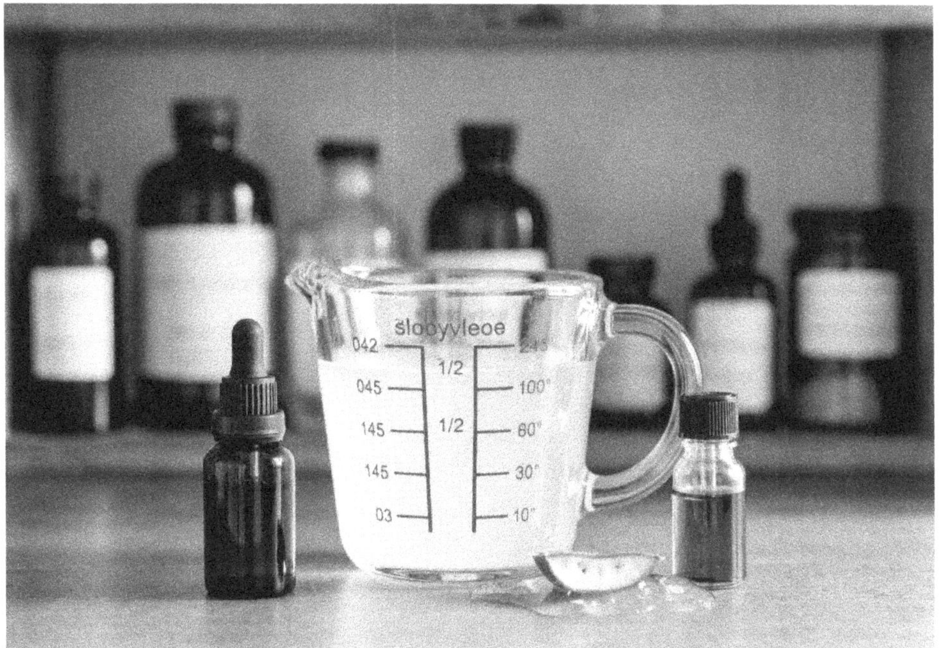

What You'll Need:

- 1/2 cup of aloe vera gel
- 10 drops of peppermint essential oil
- 5 drops of eucalyptus essential oil

Steps to Prepare:

1. Put the aloe vera gel into a clean bowl.
2. Add the peppermint and eucalyptus oils.
3. Stir everything together until it's fully combined.

Suggested Usage:

Gently rub a small amount onto areas where your skin feels irritated, repeating as often as necessary for comfort.

Important Cautions:

Skip this if your skin reacts badly to strong scents or plant-based oils; test a tiny spot first to check for any redness or discomfort.

Soothing Cucumber-Aloe Blend for Sun-Exposed Skin

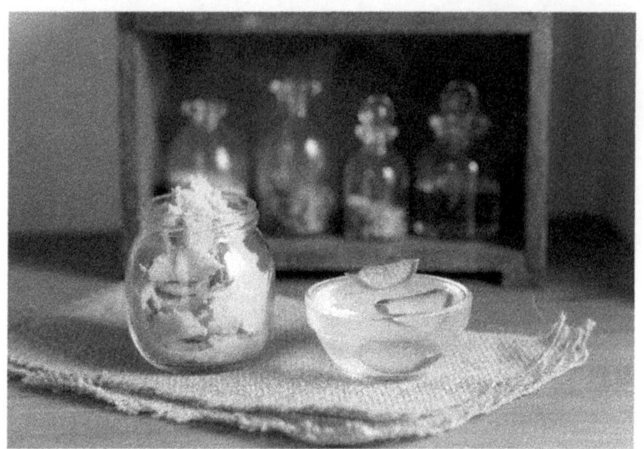

What You'll Need:

- One medium cucumber, pureed into a smooth paste
- Three tablespoons of pure aloe vera gel from the plant or a natural store-bought version

Steps to Prepare:

1. Wash the cucumber thoroughly, then chop it into pieces and puree it in a blender until it's a fine, liquid consistency.
2. In a clean bowl, combine the pureed cucumber with the aloe vera gel, stirring gently until fully blended into a light, even mixture.
3. Transfer the blend to a small jar or container for easy storage in the fridge.

Suggested Usage:

Gently spread a thin layer onto areas affected by sun exposure as needed throughout the day to help calm and refresh the skin.

Important Cautions:

Do not apply to areas with open cuts, rashes, or highly irritated skin; always test a small patch first to check for any personal sensitivity.

Soothing Blossom Brew with Natural Sweetener

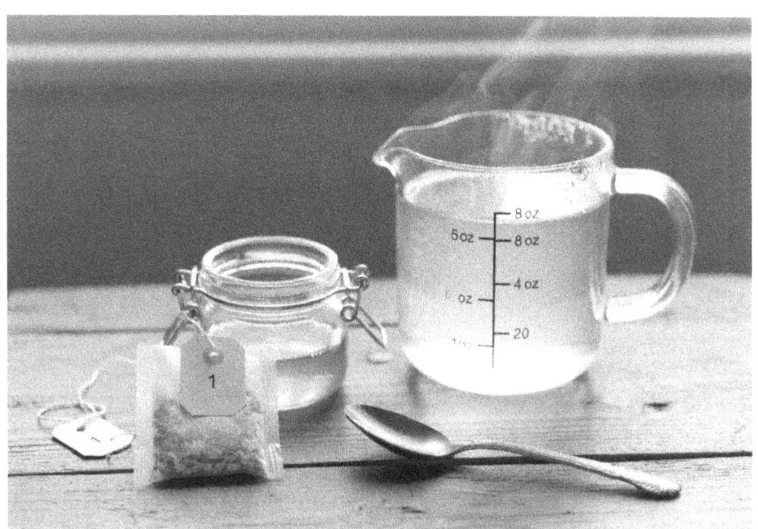

What You'll Need:

- A single packet of dried chamomile flowers (or one tea bag if preferred)
- One spoonful of pure honey
- Eight ounces of freshly boiled water

Steps to Prepare:

1. Place the chamomile in a mug and pour the boiling water over it.
2. Allow it to sit undisturbed for about five minutes to let the flavors release.
3. Mix in the honey until it fully dissolves, creating a smooth blend.

Suggested Usage:

Sip this gentle drink up to two times daily to help ease bodily swelling and promote a sense of calm.

Important Cautions:

Avoid if you are expecting a baby, as it may not be suitable during pregnancy. Always check with a healthcare provider if you have any concerns or ongoing health conditions.

Citrus Root Soothing Brew

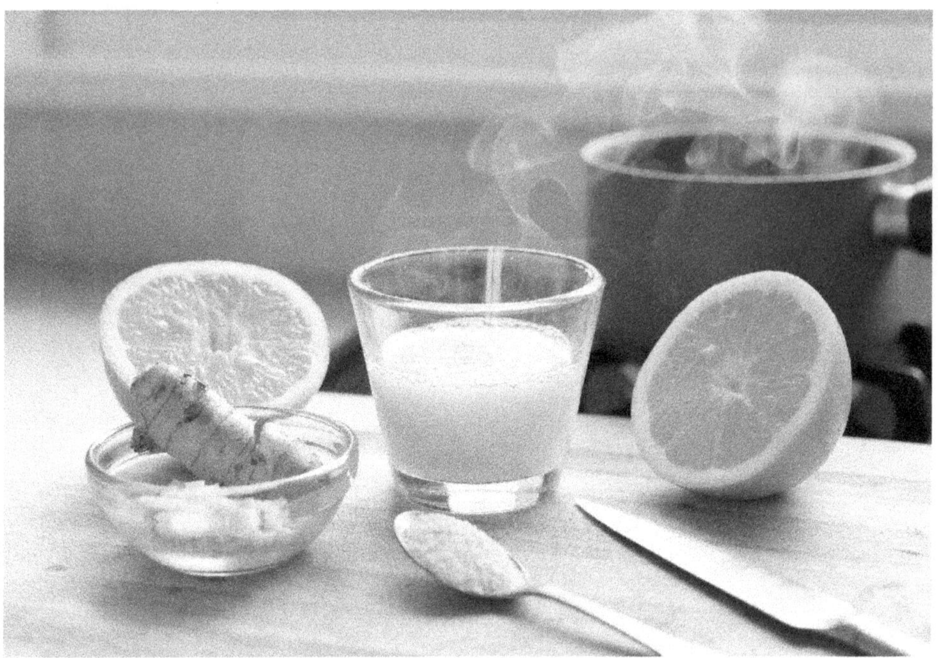

What You'll Need:

- Fresh juice from half a citrus fruit
- A small piece of peeled spice root, finely chopped (about 1/2 inch)
- 1 teaspoon of natural sweetener like agave nectar
- 8 ounces of boiling water

Steps to Prepare:

1. Pour the boiling water over the chopped spice root and let it sit for 5 minutes to infuse.
2. Mix in the citrus juice and sweetener until well blended.

Suggested Usage:

Sip this warm drink about 20 minutes prior to eating to help ease stomach discomfort and support smooth food processing.

Important Cautions:

Avoid if you often experience heartburn or stomach acid issues, as it might worsen symptoms.

Soothing Sea Salt and Floral Oil Foot Rub

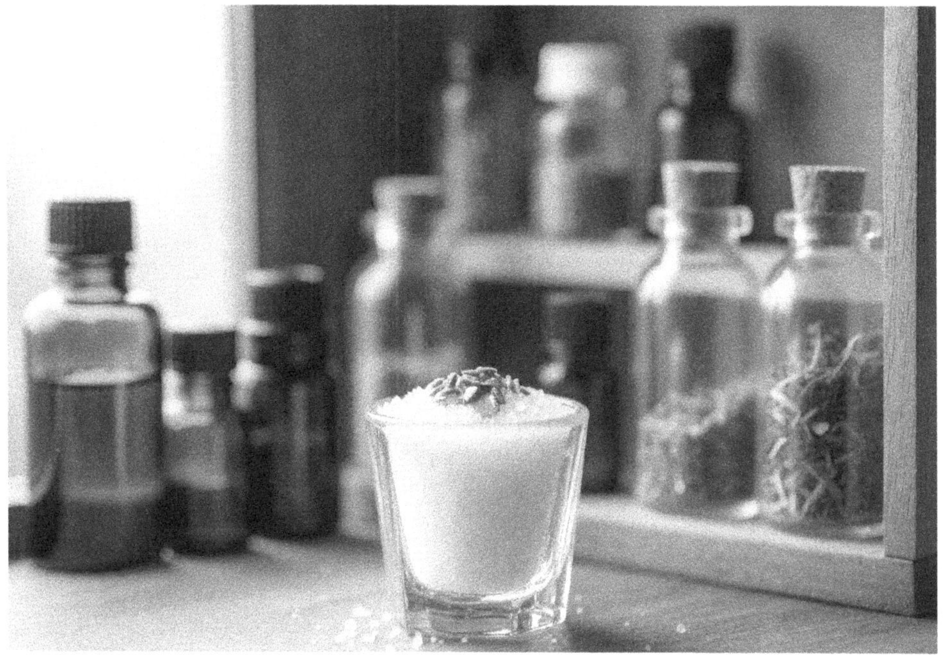

What You'll Need:

- Half a cup of sea salt (fine grain works best)
- Four drops of chamomile essential oil
- Six drops of lavender essential oil

Steps to Prepare:

1. Pour the sea salt into a small bowl.
2. Add the chamomile and lavender oils, then stir everything together until the scents blend evenly.

Suggested Usage:

Gently rub the mixture into your feet in circular motions for about five to eight minutes, ideally in the evening to help you unwind after a long day.

Important Cautions:

Steer clear of applying this if you have any breaks in the skin or irritated areas to prevent discomfort.

Warming Spice Pack for Chest Relief

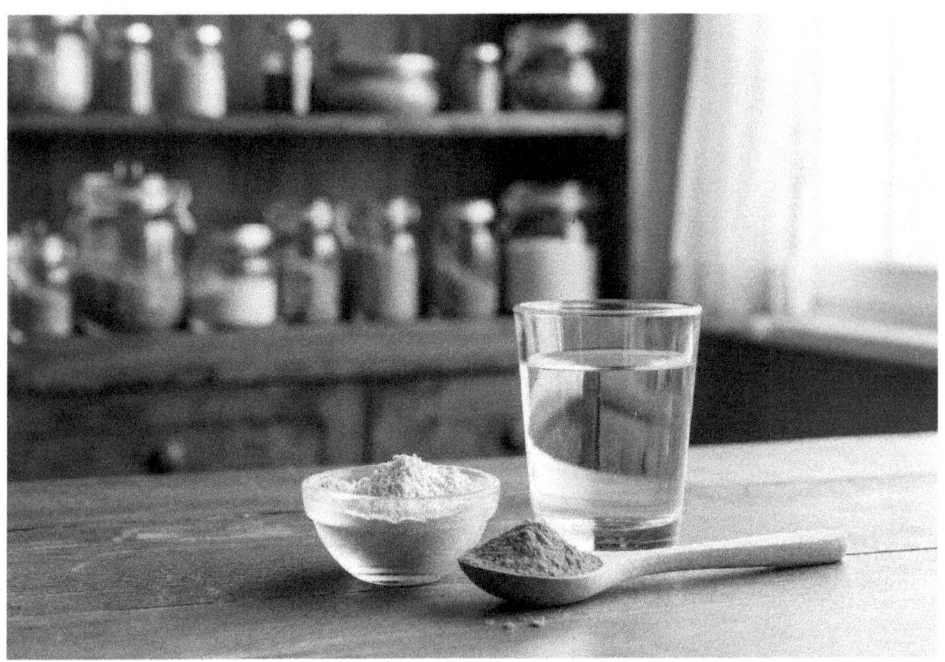

What You'll Need:

- 1 tablespoon ground ginger
- 1 teaspoon ground cinnamon
- 1/2 cup lukewarm water

Steps to Prepare:

1. Stir the ground ginger and cinnamon into the lukewarm water until fully combined.
2. Dunk a clean fabric into the blend, squeeze out extra liquid, and lay it over your chest for around 15 minutes.

Suggested Usage:

Apply it anytime you want support for easing cold discomfort.

Important Cautions:

Check that the water feels comfortably warm to prevent any skin discomfort.

Floral Hydrating Elixir for Timeless Glow

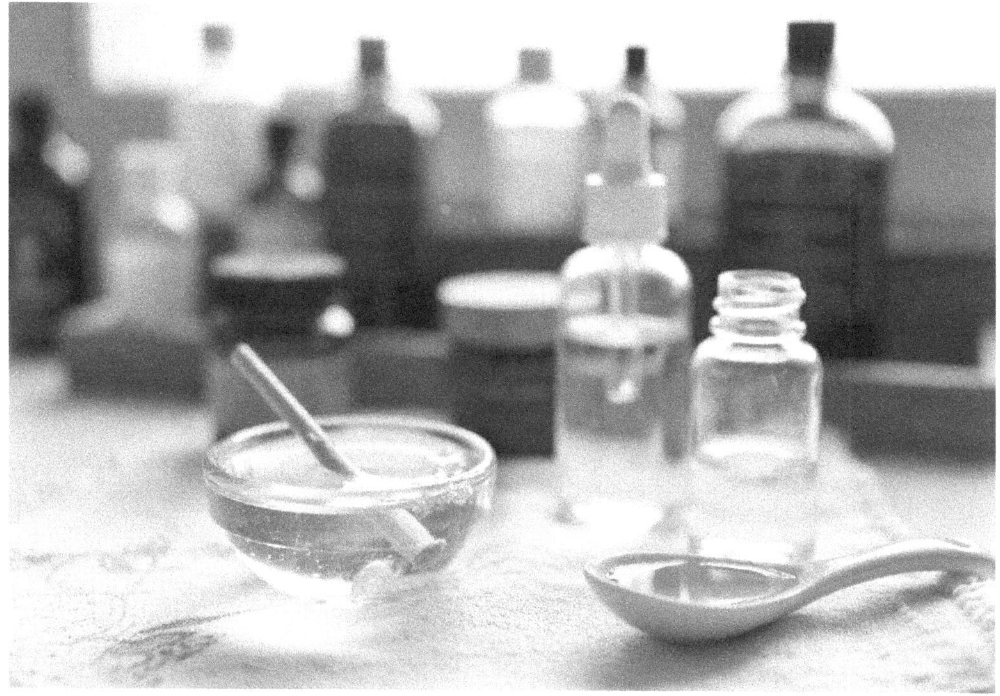

What You'll Need:

- 2 tablespoons of gentle rose-infused liquid (a soothing floral base that helps calm and refresh the skin)
- 1/2 teaspoon of natural astringent toner (like a mild herbal extract that tightens pores without drying)
- 1 tablespoon of lightweight nourishing oil (such as a plant-derived moisturizer that mimics the skin's natural barrier)

Steps to Prepare:

1. Pour the rose-infused liquid into a clean glass container with a secure lid.
2. Add the astringent toner and nourishing oil, then gently swirl or shake to blend everything evenly until it forms a smooth mixture.
3. Store in a cool, dark spot to keep it fresh for up to two weeks.

Suggested Usage:

Dab a small amount onto clean skin each evening as part of your bedtime routine to help promote a more youthful appearance over time, allowing the blend to absorb while you rest.

Important Cautions:

Always do a small patch test on your inner arm 24 hours before full application to check for any irritation or allergic reaction. Avoid contact with eyes, and discontinue use if redness or discomfort occurs. Consult a healthcare professional if you have sensitive skin conditions or are pregnant.

Veggie Glow Facial Blend

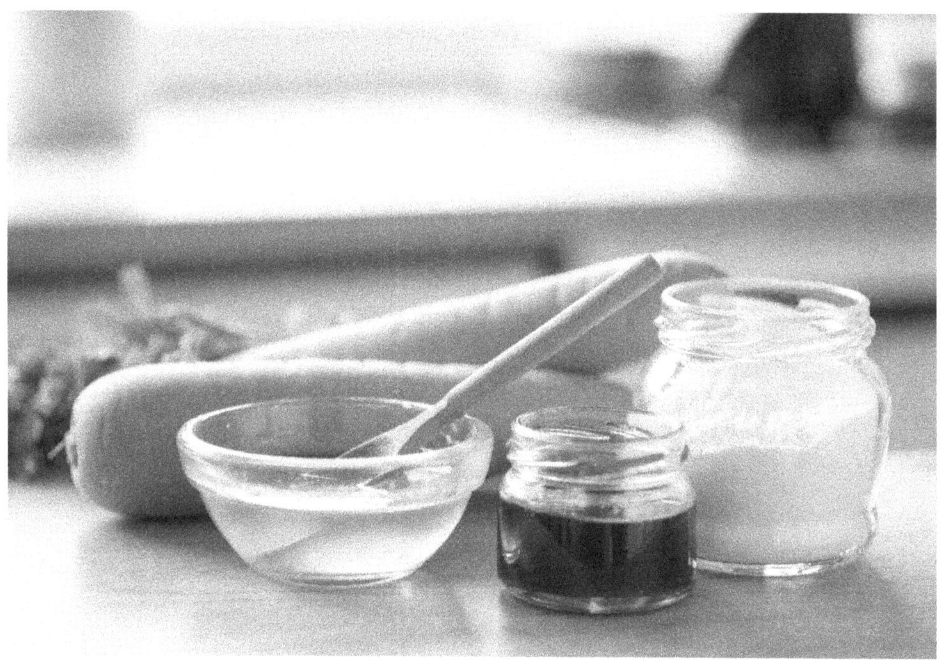

What You'll Need:

- 2 tablespoons fresh carrot juice
- 1 teaspoon raw honey
- 1 teaspoon plain milk

Steps to Prepare:

1. Combine the carrot juice, honey, and milk in a small bowl.
2. Stir until you get an even mixture.
3. Spread it gently over your clean face, avoiding the eyes.
4. Let it sit for about 10 minutes, then rinse off with cool water.

Suggested Usage:

Apply this once every seven days to help refresh and even out your skin tone.

Important Cautions:

Always do a quick check on a small spot of skin to make sure it doesn't cause any irritation before full use.

Golden Root and Citrus Skin Smoother

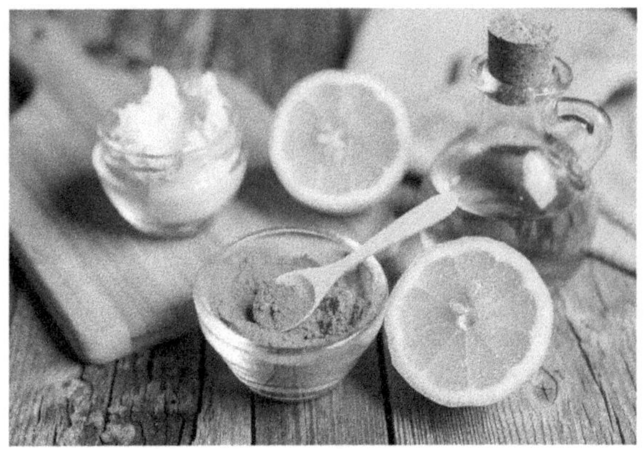

What You'll Need:

- 1 teaspoon ground golden spice (turmeric)
- 2 teaspoons fresh citrus extract (lemon squeeze)
- 3 tablespoons natural moisturizer (coconut butter)
- Optional: A dash of sweet nectar (honey) for extra soothing

Steps to Prepare:

1. Gently warm the natural moisturizer in a small bowl over low heat until it's soft and easy to blend.
2. Stir in the ground golden spice and citrus extract until everything combines into a smooth paste.
3. If using, mix in the sweet nectar for added gentleness.
4. Let the mixture cool before storing in a clean jar.

Suggested Usage:

Apply a thin layer to affected skin areas before bed, allowing it to work while you sleep. Rinse off in the morning with mild soap. Repeat each evening for gradual improvement in skin appearance.

Important Cautions:

Avoid applying to any cuts or irritated areas. This blend may temporarily tint the skin yellow, so test on a small spot first. Consult a doctor if you have sensitive skin or allergies.

Real-Life Stories from Everyday Users

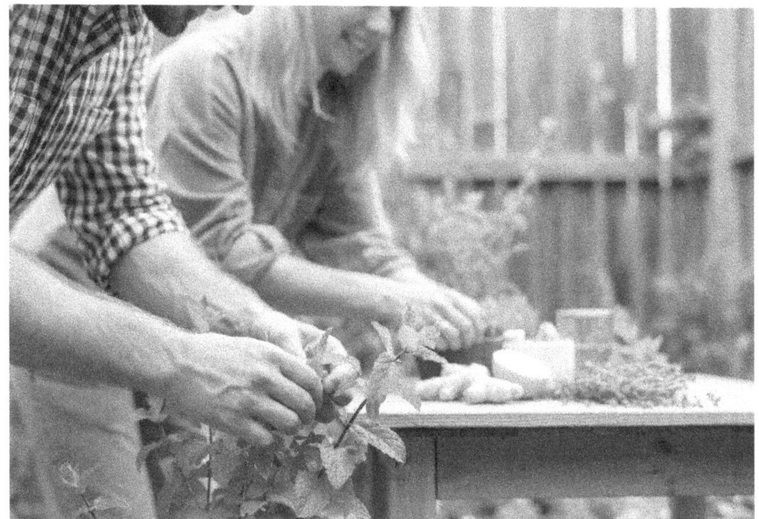

- **Peppermint Leaves for Breathing Ease**

"During hay fever season, I added peppermint leaves to hot water for a simple steam session. Right away, my airways felt clearer, and the stuffiness faded fast."

- **Ginger Root for Sore Joints** "

My aunt relies on ginger root to ease her stiff knees. She brews it into a warm drink with a touch of honey, and she finds the puffiness goes down, making movement smoother."

- **Chamomile Gel for Sun-Kissed Skin**

"Following a sunny hike, I smoothed chamomile-infused gel on my red skin. It cooled the burn instantly and toned down the irritation. Now I grow chamomile in pots at home."

- **Lavender Essence for Tension Headaches**

"Tension headaches hit me hard, but lavender essence changed that. A gentle dab on my forehead, and the tight pressure begins to lift in no time."

- **Lemon Balm Mix for Throat Comfort**

"When a scratchy throat and sniffles struck, I stirred lemon balm with warm water and a dash of citrus. It calmed my throat and helped shake off the discomfort quicker than store-bought options."

- **Fennel Seeds for Steady Energy**

"My cousin managed his energy dips after a health check by adding fennel seeds to his meals. Soon, he saw his daily vitality pick up noticeably."

- **Thyme Aroma for Sharp Thinking**

"While prepping for a big presentation, I used thyme in a room spray. It sharpened my focus, and studies suggest thyme's scent can boost mental clarity."

- **Lime Infusion for Daily Cleanse**

"I kick off each morning with lime-infused water. It's my go-to for gut health and a fresh start, leading to clearer skin and more pep in my step."

- **Ashwagandha for Vitality Boost**

"Feeling run down from busy days, I tried ashwagandha in capsule form. Within days, my stamina improved, and I tackled tasks with renewed drive."

- **Mint Slices for Tired Eyes**

"Screen time left my eyes swollen and weary. Placing fresh mint leaves over them for a short rest brought quick coolness and reduced the puff."

- **Scent Blends for Calm Days**

"To handle work pressures, I diffuse blends of rose, valerian, and bergamot. It's my way to unwind and keep worries at bay during tough times."

- **Tea Tree Extract for Gum Discomfort**

"A nagging gum ache had me worried, so I applied diluted tea tree extract. It eased the soreness fast, holding me over until my check-up."

- **Olive Oil for Stronger Locks**

"Work stress thinned my hair, but regular olive oil rubs on my scalp helped. Over time, my strands grew fuller and more vibrant."

- **Salt Scrub for Clear Skin**

"In my teen years, skin spots were a hassle, but a gentle salt and honey mix scrubbed them away, keeping my face smooth and balanced."

- **Turmeric for Travel Upset**

"On a bumpy car ride, queasiness set in. Sipping turmeric tea settled my stomach swiftly, letting me enjoy the journey."

- **Rice Soak for Itchy Patches**

"An unexpected skin flare-up itched badly, but a rice water bath soothed it right away, easing the redness without fuss."

- **Vinegar Rinse for Flaky Scalp**

"Flakes plagued my scalp for ages until I used a mild vinegar wash after shampooing. It freshened everything up and kept issues away."

- **Herbal Tea for Face Glow**

"Applying cooled herbal tea as a skin wipe transformed my routine. The natural boosters cut down on spots and evened my tone."

- **Plant Jelly for Scalp Care**

"Dry scalp made my hair dull, but plant-based jelly treatments nourished it deeply, leaving locks soft and flake-free without strong products."

- **Banana Blend for Skin Hydration**

"For years, I've mashed banana with yogurt for a quick face treatment. It locks in moisture, leaving my skin smooth and refreshed."

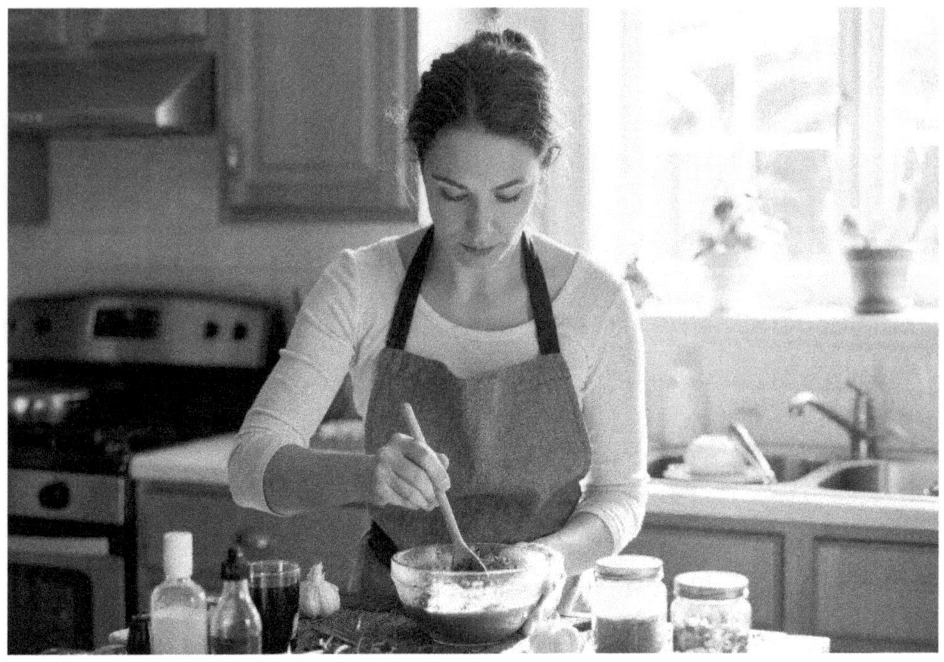

As the author, I'm truly grateful for the chance to pass along the tips and natural fixes you'll find here. While building and fine-tuning this guide, I've blended my life stories, careful studies, and time-tested ideas to create a well-rounded resource for everyday wellness. Every suggestion draws from real evidence and my hands-on adventures in staying healthy the natural way.

The review stage went beyond just fixing words—it focused on making sure each tip is straightforward, doable, and truly helpful for anyone looking to boost their own health. Whether tweaking the style or double-checking facts, I've shaped every part with a single aim: to help you steer your well-being using simple, nature-based methods.

By mixing in a variety of tips and ways to use them, I've worked to build a full handbook that fits right into your personal path to feeling better. Now that it's all wrapped up, I truly wish the positive changes and fresh starts you discover through these ideas are only the start. Thanks so much for coming along on this journey toward stronger, self-guided health.

www.ingramcontent.com/pod-product-compliance
Lightning Source LLC
Chambersburg PA
CBHW040934070726

47599CB00036B/1844